Physical Medicine and Rehabilitation

Clinics of North America

Consulting Editor

George H. Kraft, MD

Guest Editors

Michael T. Andary, MD, and
Mark A. Tomski, MD

OFFICE MANAGEMENT OF PAIN

FEBRUARY 1993

W.B. SAUNDERS COMPANY
Harcourt Brace Jovanovich, Inc.

Philadelphia • London • Toronto • Montreal • Sydney • Tokyo

W. B. SAUNDERS COMPANY
Harcourt Brace Jovanovich, Inc.

The Curtis Center
Independence Square West
Philadelphia, PA 19106–3399

Physical Medicine and Rehabilitation Clinics is indexed in *Cumulative Index to Nursing and Allied Health Literature.*

PHYSICAL MEDICINE AND REHABILITATION CLINICS OF NORTH AMERICA

February 1993   **Volume 4, Number 1**   **ISSN 1047–9651**

The following information is published in accordance with the requirements of the United States Postal Code.

The *Physical Medicine and Rehabilitation Clinics of North America* (ISSN 1047–9651) is published four times yearly by the W. B. Saunders Company. Corporate and Editorial Offices: The Curtis Center, Independence Square West, Philadelphia, PA 19106–3399. Accounting and Circulation Offices: 6277 Sea Harbor Drive, Orlando, FL 32887-4800. Second-class postage paid at Orlando, FL 32887, and additional mailing offices. Subscription price is $73.00 per year (U.S. individuals), $89.00 (U.S. institutions), and $101.00 (foreign). Foreign air speed delivery for all *Clinics* is $8.00 per issue. All prices are subject to change without notice. POSTMASTER: Send address changes to *Physical Medicine and Rehabilitation Clinics of North America* (ISSN 1047–9651), W. B. Saunders Company, Periodicals Fulfillment, Orlando, FL 32887-4800.

Customer Service: 1-800-654-2452

The editor of this publication is Kelly Thomas, W. B. Saunders Company, The Curtis Center, Independence Square West, Philadelphia, PA 19106-3399.

CONSULTING EDITOR

GEORGE H. KRAFT, MD, Professor, Department of Rehabilitation Medicine, Chief of Staff-Elect, University of Washington Medical Center; Director, Electrodiagnostic Medicine, Multiple Sclerosis Clinical Center, Muscular Dystrophy Clinical Center, University of Washington, Seattle, Washington

GUEST EDITORS

MICHAEL T. ANDARY, MD, Associate Professor, Department of Physical Medicine and Rehabilitation, Michigan State University College of Osteopathic Medicine, East Lansing, Michigan

MARK A. TOMSKI, MD, Clinical Assistant Professor, Department of Rehabilitation Medicine, University of Washington, Seattle; and Private Practice, Puyallup, Washington

CONTRIBUTORS

MICHAEL T. ANDARY, MD, Associate Professor, Department of Physical Medicine and Rehabilitation, Michigan State University College of Osteopathic Medicine, East Lansing, Michigan

RANDY BAKER, RA, Research Associate, Department of Orthopaedics, University of Washington, Seattle, Washington

STANLEY J. BIGOS, MD, Professor of Orthopaedic Surgery and Occupational Health, and Director, Spine Resource Clinic, University of Washington, Seattle, Washington

MICHAEL C. BRODY, MD, Department of Anesthesiology, The Medical Center, Beaver, Pennsylvania

F. PETER BUCKLEY, MB, FFARCS, Associate Professor, Department of Anesthesiology, and Attending Physician, Multidisciplinary Pain Clinic, University of Washington School of Medicine; and Medical Director, Pain and Toxicity Program, Fred Hutchinson Cancer Research Center, Seattle, Washington

iii

CHARLES CHABAL, MD, Assistant Professor, Department of Anesthesiology, and Attending Physician, Multidisciplinary Pain Clinic, University of Washington School of Medicine; and Veterans Administration Medical Center, Seattle, Washington

THOMAS B. CORSOLINI, PT, MD, Private Practice, Corvallis, Oregon

PETER C. ESSELMAN, MD, Assistant Professor, Department of Rehabilitation Medicine, University of Washington, Seattle, Washington

PHILIP E. GREENMAN, MD, Professor, Departments of Biomechanics and Physical Medicine and Rehabilitation, Michigan State University College of Osteopathic Medicine, East Lansing, Michigan

ANDREW J. HAIG, MD, Medical Director, The Center for Rehabilitation Services, Theda Clark Regional Medical Center, Neenah; and Clinical Assistant Professor, Department of Physical Medicine and Rehabilitation, Medical College of Wisconsin, Milwaukee, Wisconsin

SID LEE, RA, Research Associate, UCLA Emergency Medical Center, Los Angeles, California

CHARLES C. MAULDIN, Jr, MD, Medical Director of Rehabilitation Services, Cox Medical Centers, Springfield, Missouri

MICHEL LACERTE, MDCM, MSc, FRCPC, Assistant Professor, Department of Physical Medicine and Rehabilitation, and Director, Disability Evaluation Program, University of Western Ontario, London, Ontario, Canada

JAY MEYTHALER, JD, MD, Associate Professor, Spain Rehabilitation Center, Department of Rehabilitation Medicine, University of Alabama School of Medicine, Birmingham, Alabama

JOSE L. OCHOA, MD, PhD, DSc, Director, Neuromuscular Disease Unit, Good Samaritan Hospital and Medical Center; and Professor of Neurology, Oregon Health Sciences University, Portland, Oregon

JONATHAN L. RITSON, MD, Medical Director, Northwest Therapy Spine Program, Tacoma, Washington

NORMAN B. ROSEN, MD, Medical Director, Rehabilitation and Pain Management Associates of Baltimore, Baltimore, Maryland

C. NORMAN SHEALY, MD, PhD, Private Practitioner, Shealy Institute, Springfield, Missouri

DONALD F. STANTON, DO, Professor and Acting Chairman, Department of Physical Medicine and Rehabilitation, Michigan State University College of Osteopathic Medicine, East Lansing, Michigan

MARK A. TOMSKI, MD, Clinical Assistant Professor, Department of Rehabilitation Medicine, University of Washington, Seattle; and Private Practice, Puyallup, Washington

CONTRIBUTORS

RENATO J. VERDUGO, MD, Visiting Professor, Department of Neurology, Oregon Health Sciences University and Good Samaritan Hospital and Medical Center, Portland, Oregon; and Associate Professor, Department of Neurological Sciences, Faculty of Medicine, University of Chile, Santiago, Chile

FREDERICK VINCENT, MD, Clinical Professor of Medicine (Neurology) and Psychiatry, Michigan State University College of Human Medicine, and Clinical Professor of Internal Medicine (Neurology), Michigan State University College of Osteopathic Medicine, East Lansing, Michigan

DANIEL V. VOISS, MS, MD, Medical Director, ACCESS Consulting Systems Incorporated, Portland, Oregon

FORTHCOMING ISSUES

PREVIOUS ISSUES

CONTENTS

organ of adaptation is underscored; we are our brains, and brain, body, and mind are one.

Myofascial Pain Syndromes

Norman B. Rosen

Over the past 10 to 15 years, there has been a significant increase in our understanding of those diseases of the musculoskeletal system that cause muscular pain and dysfunction. Chief among them are the myofascial pain syndromes, which continue to be among the most overlooked and undertreated causes of musculoskeletal pain and dysfunction. This review explores some of the controversial aspects of our understanding of the muscle pain syndromes and reviews the critical components of evaluating and treating any patient who presents with myofascial pain and dysfunction. There is a need for a common terminology among the various disciplines that deal with patients who present with musculoskeletal pain and dysfunction, and a clasification of muscle pain disorders is proposed. There are also needs to understand where the myofascial pain syndromes fit in the broader group of disorders involving both muscle and joint and to approach the patient simultaneously from two divergent perspectives, exploring dysfunction at the tissue level and dysfunction relative to the interaction of the patient with and in his or her environment.

Legal Issues Involved in the Outpatient Management of Pain

Jay Meythaler

Legal issues confront the physician frequently when he or she deals with patients in the outpatient management of pain. These issues involve proper documentation for establishing disability with regard to workers' compensation, the Social Security Administration, or third-party liability cases. One must also be knowledgeable about when and how to deliver proper information as an expert witness. In this article, the elements of malpractice and other causes of legal liabilities are reviewed, both to inform the physician better about the legal process and to aid him or her in steering clear of creating a legal cause of action. Finally, some issues regarding documentation for reimbursement are reviewed.

Medication and the Office Management of Pain

F. Peter Buckley and Charles Chabal

A wide variety of analgesic drugs is available to treat the pain problems encountered in a physical medicine and rehabilitation office practice. The pharmacology and indications for the use of these drugs are described in this article. The place of many of the drugs for pain management is currently controversial. Analgesics should be used for specific purposes and targeted at specific nociceptive problems.

sponse to these procedures, which in the case of sympathetic blocks has engendered the concept of sympathetically maintained pain (SMP), is most likely the expression of active placebo effect. Although animal models of nerve injury do provide important data on abnormal peripheral and central nervous system dysfunction, such discrete models misrepresent the broad clinical conditions of RSD-SMP. The issue is futher complicated by all-embracing definitions that retain the word *sympathetic*. Revision of current theories to explain RSD-SMP, and procedures to diagnose and attempt to treat these patients, are well overdue.

Many different treatments are available for reflex sympathetic dystrophy. Treatment of the precipitating cause and increases in physical activity are the cornerstones of therapy. Regional blocks, systemic medications, or electrostimulation in combination with therapy offers the most common modalities for primary initial treatment. The earlier treatment is instituted, the better the response. Nonphysical, psychological, and vocational factors need to be considered in every patient, and multidisciplinary and interdisciplinary team treatment may be necessary.

Historically, electrotherapeutics has been within the purview of charlatans, but evidence that some modern techniques may have specific therapeutic benefit for pain is emerging. Both commonly used and promising newer devices or techniques are discussed in this article, with emphasis on practical application.

Patients with persistent (chronic) pain often undergo repeated diagnostic efforts and are treated with multiple, ineffective treatment regimens. Unnecessary suffering and disability too often result. Dealing with these issues can be facilitated by proper understanding of the disorder and with knowledge of the types of pain clinics available and what to expect from each.

FOREWORD

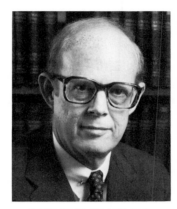

GEORGE H. KRAFT, MD
Consulting Editor

This issue of the *Physical Medicine and Rehabilitation Clinics of North America* marks the first issue of 1993 and the second volume with co–Guest Editors. Its emphasis is on the outpatient management of chronic pain, which has become an important part of physiatric practice, in most cases managed in the office. Many, if not most, chronic pain problems originate from musculoskeletal sources. Medication, the issue of pain versus disability, the approach to facilitating return to work, sympathetic pain problems, use of modalities, manual techniques, and legal issues involved, as well as other areas, are all covered in this issue. Therefore, it is fitting that this issue has Guest Editors who bring together the experience of the University of Washington, the institution that originated the pain clinic concept, and Michigan State University, the major osteopathic medical school in America.

I was pleased when Drs. Andary and Tomski agreed to guest edit this issue. Dr. Tomski is on the clinical faculty of the Department of Rehabilitation Medicine at the University of Washington, and Dr. Andary, having developed an outpatient chronic pain program at the University of Washington, is currently on the faculty of the College of Osteopathic Medicine at Michigan State University. Most physiatrists with whom I've talked regarding musculoskeletal pain feel that manual medicine is an area often neglected in their training programs. Consequently, the perspective of Dr. Andary on this topic is greatly anticipated.

There are some especially well known contributors to this issue: Dr. Peter Buckley of the University of Washington's Pain Clinic; Dr. Stanley Bigos, Director of the University of Washington Spine Resources Center; Dr. Philip Greenman, prolific writer and teacher of osteopathic manual medicine; Dr. Norman Shealy of the Shealy Institute; and Dr. José Ochoa, a well known investigator in the area of peripheral nerve dysfunction, to name just a few. Other contributors to this issue are Drs. Andrew Haig, Michel Lacerte, Daniel Voiss, Norman Rosen, Jay Meythaler, Charles Chabal, Jonathan Ritson, Frederick Vincent, Peter Esselman, Renato Verdugo, Michael Brody, Charles Mauldin, Donald Stanton, and Thomas Corsolini, as well as Randy Baker and Sid Lee. The authors are from institutions specializing in chronic pain management in the United States and Canada, fitting for a *Clinics* of North America! Drs. Andary and Tomski have done a superb job of recruiting colleagues and organizing an impressive and useful contribution to the physician's library.

GEORGE H. KRAFT, MD
Consulting Editor

Department of Rehabilitation Medicine, RJ-30
University of Washington School of Medicine
BB919 Health Science Building
1959 N. E. Pacific Street
Seattle, WA 98195

PREFACE

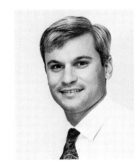 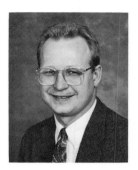

MICHAEL T. ANDARY, MD   MARK A. TOMSKI, MD
Guest Editors

When George H. Kraft, MD, offered us the opportunity of putting together this issue on the outpatient management of pain, we decided early that there is no way to cover all aspects of pain reasonably. We chose instead to select topics that are of some general interest, are important for the management of patients with pain, and may not necessarily have had widespread exposure in the rehabilitation literature.

It will be readily apparent that there are many different and often conflicting viewpoints expressed in this issue. We make no attempt to resolve those differences definitively but rather present them so readers can decide for themselves. There appear to be several unifying tenets of treatment that we do think important, and they include:

1. Patients who present to physicians with pain complaints do so for many reasons, and it is important that the physician look beyond the simple pain complaints to recognize other organic, psychological, social, or environmental problems that are contributing to the pain behaviors.
2. It is important to use medications and therapies appropriately to encourage early increase in activity and return to work, thus avoiding problems encountered in the development of the chronic pain syndrome.
3. It is still incumbent on physicians to advocate for their patients; to do so often requires an understanding of the social, administrative, and legal systems that affect them.
4. Physicians need to recognize that there comes a time when they will no longer be able to treat the pain and must therefore modify their goals to improve patient function.
5. Physicians should continue to be involved in the modification of the administrative and legal systems to allow more appropriate medical care of our patients.

An effort was made to make this a conceptual volume, versus a cookbook, to aid the clinician in treating these most challenging patients in new and creative ways.

xiii

We would like to offer our heartfelt thanks to Dr. Kraft for the opportunity of working with him on this volume of *Physical Medicine and Rehabilitation Clinics of North America.*

MICHAEL T. ANDARY, MD
MARK A. TOMSKI, MD
Guest Editors

Department of Physical Medicine and Rehabilitation
College of Osteopathic Medicine
Michigan State University
B-401 West Fee Hall
East Lansing, MI 48824-1316

7329 18th Avenue, NW
Seattle, WA 98117

THE BUSINESS OF DISSOCIATING PAIN AND DISABILITIES

Andrew J. Haig, MD

Pain and disability are not always related. It is sometimes depressing that so many people come into my office with pain and leave with the same pain. Often when they do thank me for the relief of their pain, in my heart I know that time was the cure and I have taken the credit. Occasionally, I even make their pain worse by recommending a painful diagnostic or treatment modality. Despite all the successful treatments described in this issue and other publications, the fact is that when all is said and done, my hands are often tied when it comes to relief of the patient's pain.

On the other hand, disability is something I can almost always do something about. Counseling, exercise, equipment, job modification, education—hardly a person leaves my office without some tools to allow him or her to perform the enjoyable and necessary activities of life that he or she had given up. Sometimes, when the disability is removed, the pain just is not so important anymore. I can feel proud that most patients' lives are changed for the better if I treat their disability.

This issue is about pain: diagnosis, quantification, and treatment in an office setting. It is also about disability related to pain. It is very appropriate that one article deal with disability alone. To treat pain alone when disability exists is a therapeutic oversight. To allow a program for pain actually to interfere with recovery from disability is counter to the patients' interests unless that program has a very high rate of complete cure.

In this article we discuss the management of disability in the office practice of physicians who treat pain. The goal of this article is not to outline treatment protocols for the many different painful and disabling conditions. That task has been accomplished in this issue and others. Instead, we focus on the practice style itself. A theme of the article is the use of proven business techniques to our

From the Center for Rehabilitation Services, Theda Clark Regional Medical Center, Neenah; and Department of Physical Medicine and Rehabilitation, Medical College of Wisconsin, Milwaukee, Wisconsin patient's benefit. First, we present a "sales" interviewing style that establishes patient expectations regarding function. Next, we address the prevention of iatrogenic disability by eliminating production quotas. Finally, we illustrate ways in which our practice can measure and improve the quality of its "product" by streamlining the assembly process and implementing a quality-assurance program.

THE ESSENCE OF SALES: ANTICIPATING PATIENT NEEDS

"Hi, I'm Dr. Haig. Are you John?" "Yes." "Where do you come from?" "Oshkosh. Well, I actually grew up in Milwaukee." "What do you like to do outside of work?" "I used to like to fish, but now that my back hurts, I can't do anything." "Oh. We'll talk more about your back in a few minutes. Tell me more about you. What did you like to do before your injury?" "I did everything . . . you know . . . ." "Everything? Like what?" "I fished sometimes." "Fished? Where?" "Last year I got a 14-foot Boston Whaler with a 20 hp Johnson and my buddy and I go out walleye fishing every weekend to Waupaca." "Neat! I never really tried walleye fishing."

Later: "Well, John, your kind of back problem is pretty likely to go away. It's not dangerous. You should see some improvement in the next few days. Let's get you scheduled for back school. In the meantime, let's figure out some ways to get you back to work despite the pain you're having . . . and be sure to ask the OT about ways to sit comfortably while fishing."

Are you a salesman? Salesmen will tell you that the first few seconds of an interview make or break the deal. In the protocol used in our institution, the first words out of a physician's mouth after introduction deal with function, not pain. By asking about outside activities, the physician established his interest in the patient as a whole person, not just in the relation of the job to the injury. Redirecting the patient when he wants to jump ahead emphasizes this interest in the whole person. A patient who cannot be redirected away from the pain or cannot focus on his life outside of work may have psychosocial factors that require exploration.

The introductory questioning into the patient's avocation ends when the patient not only answers a question but elaborates, increases eye contact, or expresses some other body language indicating that he or she is discussing an area of personal importance. A remark that shows respect or interest serves as a transition to more traditional history and physical examination. The physician closes the patient visit by reinforcing the positive prognosis (if appropriate) and reminding the patient that goals of treatment include elimination of both work and avocational disabilities.

Well, are you a salesman? Such interview techniques may seen unnatural at first. In reality, it is the office setting itself that is unnatural. Twemlow and Gabbard's[8] treatise on iatrogenic illnesses states that "any kind of medical specialization involves a form of counter-transference which may result in scotomata for the patient's personhood. Thus, the patient often feels infantilized and depersonified. His reaction may be regression or undue passivity in compliance." Although many nonpsychiatrists view the patient interview as a one-way street, it is unavoidably both a therapeutic and diagnostic event. A carefully structured interview serves a dual purpose of providing diagnostic clues and developing the format of the physician–patient relationship. When there is disability related to pain, patient ownership to therapeutic goals and expectations is best developed prior to a diagnostic evaluation.

Unfortunately for physiatrists, many patients are initially seen in the chronic stage. They arrive in our office after weeks and months of unwitting or willful indoctrination by practitioners, advertisements, and society about the absolute relation between pain and function. Some patients actually make a genuine effort to "ignore the pain," and fail. Still other patients have misperceptions about the risk of neurologic damage or permanently worsened pain with activity. There is also a small group who use pain as a subconscious (hysterical) protection against activities that they wish to avoid and an even smaller group who might be malingering.

The initial few moments of the interview are crucial for the chronic group as well. The trick, as in sales, is to be prepared. Often, notes from referring physicians indicate the patient's mind-set. An intake questionnaire that includes inquiries into the patient's perception is useful. "What do you think the problem is?" "How is your boss getting along with you now?" "Before the injury?" "Aside from your pain, what is the most stressful thing in your life?"

With chronic-pain patients, we always open with the stream of questioning described earlier but quickly cut to a more leading question. The choice of question depends in part on the data that we have gathered. One important question is "What would you do differently if you finally concluded that this pain would never go away?" Some answers have profound effect on our treatment.

"I would kill myself."
"I'd quit the foundry and finish my last three credits towards my accounting
   degree."
"I guess I'd just have to bite the bullet and get back to work."
"I'd stay home and play with my baby," with a smile.

Many patients do not really answer the question, at least in terms of a life plan. Their answers also suggest certain treatment choices.

"Someone damn well better fix me."
"I'd sue the company."
"I don't even want to think about it."
"I don't know. . . . I've thought about it a lot and I really don't know. . . .
   I need the cash. I've always worked there, all of my friends are there, and
   I'm only 5 years from retirement."
"It will get better."

After such answers the physician persists until the patient provides his or her concept of the worst-case scenario. It is crucial to ask these questions early, not only to set the tone for the visit but also to avoid miscommunication. Asking such questions of chronic-pain patients after the history of present illness or physical examination has been completed might suggest that, on the basis of your examination, you think that they will never get better.

QUOTA SYSTEMS: HOW DOCTORS CAUSE DISABILITY

Physicians get thrust into impossible situations:

The patient has undergone a L4–S1 fusion. Can she lift 50 pounds?
A patient's left hand turns red and swells, and the pain is 9 on a scale of 10
   when he plays the piano. How long should he play before he stops?

W.E. Deming is well known to the business world as the man who revolutionized the Japanese economy after World War II.[7] His concepts are becoming very popular with American business and are even finding their way into health care.[5] He suggests that production quotas actually lower productivity. They allow top employees to accept mediocrity but do little to change the reasons for poor performance by others.

What does Deming have to do with pain? I wish that the facts and the questions in our examples matched up, but they do not. The answer to each of these questions is probably, "I don't know; please tell me more." Simply protecting the patient's back, or arm, or leg, without understanding the details of the task or realizing the physical, emotional, and social consequences, is contrary to the holistic approach physiatrists espouse for other people with disabilities. Yet, for our patients with pain, we often have preconceived notions of the relation between pain, pathology, personal preference, and performance. We are often requested by the employer, insurer, or the patient to place a quota on the patient's performance.

We can improve functional outcome by optimizing function. Risks can be accepted. The back-injured woman is a single mother, a former weightlifter who needs to lift a 55-lb weight twice a day from one waist-high table to another to keep her well-paying job. The piano player with reflex sympathetic dystrophy believes that his music is his life. He would gladly live with the pain as long as we can assure him that movement will not cause him to become paralyzed. If we take time truly to understand the work or avocational need and to outline the risks to our best knowledge, many patients may choose to work or play despite pain.

Risks can be modified. A wheeled platform eliminates the need for our first patient to lift. Our musician might find acceptable pieces that require fewer chords to be played with his left hand. Exercise, surgery, braces, education, task modification, environmental design, psychological therapy, relaxation techniques, and medications all can modify the pain of an activity.

Certainly, there are times when the law, bureaucracy, or real risk of substantial harm to self or others requires us to place a restriction. Patient restrictions, either written, spoken, or implied by the physician, carry a heavy weight, especially for patients who have been made to feel "infantilized."[8] Physicians need to gather a lot of information about both benefits and risks if they are to accept the responsibility of imposing their value system on their patient. In reality, physicians often do not know or do not inform patients of the real magnitude of a risk. For example, the risk of permanent impairment or neurologic deficit due to return to work with nonradiating back pain is extremely small, but the benefits of early activation are praised.[1, 6]

EFFICIENT WIDGET MAKING: ASSURING THE QUALITY OF YOUR PROGRAM

How many people talk to the patient before the psysiatrist sees a patient with simple acute low back pain in the office 2 days after injury? About 27 in our practice. Take a look at Table 1. There is a lot of repetition, waiting, and contradictory information. A lot could go wrong. No wonder our "manufacturing" process is so time-inefficient, costly, and variable in outcome. By looking at the whole process, not just his or her part in it, the physiatrist can improve quality of care.

The consulting firm Booz Allen & Hamilton studied many other hospital processes and found similar duplication and inefficiencies.[4] The result was radical restructuring of a number of major hospitals toward "patient-focused care." For instance, patients are greeted in the lobby of the hospital and escorted directly to their room, where admission paperwork, laboratory work, and nurs-

Table 1. PEOPLE INVOLVED IN THE FIRST 48 HOURS OF A SIMPLE BACK INJURY

Person	Role
Co-worker	Helps patient get up, calls the boss.
Boss-supervisor	Assesses severity. Sends to the plant nurse.
Plant nurse	Assesses severity again. Sends to emergency room.
Company driver or ambulance	Drives to emergency room (driver is on light duty).
Admitting secretary	Asks whether this is a workmen's compensation case. Gets signature.
Emergency room nurse	Assesses severity. Checks vital signs.
Emergency room physician	Assesses severity. Decides on radiography.
Emergency room aide	Transports to x-ray unit in a wheelchair.
X-ray scheduler	Tells patient where to wait. Decides how long.
X-ray technologist	Takes radiograph.
Radiologist	Reads radiograph. Dictates note.
X-ray transcriptionist	Transcribes. Sends results to physical medicine and rehabilitation (maybe).
X-ray aide	Transports back to emergency room.
Emergency room nurse (new shift)	Checks to be sure patient is back. Notifies physician.
Emergency room physician (new shift)	Discusses results, restrictions, treatment.
Emergency room nurse (new shift)	Reviews discharge instructions.
Emergency room secretary	Schedules physical medicine and rehabilitation appointment.
Emergency room transcriptionist	Transcribes. Sends results to physical medicine and rehabilitation (maybe).
Pharmacist	Fills prescription.
Plant driver	Drives patient home.
Spouse	Assesses severity. Keeps kids quiet for a change.
Fishing partner	Assesses severity. Suggests his chiropractor.
Boss-supervisor	Reports in sick. Suggests Doan's Pills.
Company nurse	Reinforces emergency room plan. Explains workmen's compensation.
Physical medicine and rehabilitation secretary	Schedules, assembles records, registers.
Physical medicine and rehabilitation nurse	Assesses severity. Reviews data and vitals.
Physiatrist	"Hi, I'm Dr. Haig. Are you John?"

ing evaluation are done by the same person. X-ray facilities and satellite laboratories are on the same floor. The transport aide also does the job of phlebotomist, unit secretary, and medical records clerk.

Few physician practices would hire a consultant to study management of the component of their practice that deals with pain, because it involves too much time and money. We can easily copy Booz Allen's approach, however. Find one group of pain patients whose care is of concern: chronic back pain, shoulder-hand syndrome, repetitive trauma disorder, whatever. Map out the process that patients go through during the care of their pain. Make it as specific and locally relevant as possible. Begin with causes for the illness, reasons the patient seeks attention, reasons for choosing certain practitioners, and reasons the patient arrives in your practice. Identify as many people, resources, treatment options, delays and variations that affect the patient as possible. Be sure to include factors outside the practice that influence the treatment. Identify other people with a stake in the management of the patient. Many of the changes needed to stream-line the process become obvious.

With a better understanding of the whole process, creative problem solving can reduce risk, cost, and confusion for the patient. For instance, in the example of acute low back pain, we met with the emergency-room physicians, nurses, and secretaries to explain the process. Together, we agreed that the emergency room would share a part of our questionnaire as an intake data base. Nurses, having learned the good prognosis for most patients, developed a more positive-sounding back-pain information booklet. Thus, patients were less anxious and less likely to be confused by unsolicited and inaccurate advice. Physicians under-stood that we would accept responsibility for a diagnostic work-up, so radio-graphs were less likely to be ordered on initial visit. Secretaries met with our office staff to ensure that appropriate data were forwarded and in turn asked for open appointment times to avoid phone hassles. We all made a renewed effort to communicate consistently with the employer to minimize disability.

Pain specialists may debate over the validity of most specific medical treat-ments. That argument aside, few would disagree that unnecessary delays in return to work or activity worsen prognosis. Still, not many take a calculated look at elimination of hassles, ambiguity, waiting, and duplication in the process of treatment. The Booz Allen approach is one way to do so.

Our patients are not widgets! It's true. A hallmark of good practice is individ-ualized consideration of each patient. The industrialist Deming couldn't agree more. Actually a statistician, he insisted that, even in industry, variation cannot be eliminated. By understanding variation and its causes, Deming demonstrated that improvements in the system could be made.[2] For instance, one worker in a manufacturing plant might perform worse than average during one quarter. The supervisor is tempted to place the worker on probation or change his methods; however, if on further data collection that worker's performance falls within two standard deviations of the norm, most likely this worker is randomly performing within the system. To punish or change this employee is just as likely to harm as to help. Left alone, he might be the top performer during the next quarter. While performances that fall out of two standard deviations are studied to find out what went wrong or right, the system as a whole must change to make system-wide improvements. In one medical model, McEachern and others[5] have demon-strated that the Deming approach to continuous quality improvement (CQI) resulted in a drastic decline in the number of cesarean sections.

How does CQI work? The first step is to identify the customers and their needs. Despite our primary concern for the patient, there are many other individ-uals who must be viewed as customers because they can have a profound effect on the outcome of an individual case as well as the scope of referrals to our office practice. Their needs do not all have to be respected, but do need to be under-stood. Table 2 lists typical customers in a case of work-related pain.

Deming speaks of exceeding customer expectation, which means that we need to understand the real, not just the spoken, needs of our customers. The second step is to define these needs. By interviewing a few key customers expressly for understanding their needs, we can learn how these customers can affect functional outcome for our primary customer, the patient. Table 2 suggests some typical needs, spoken and unspoken, of the various customers.

Next, we need to measure outcome based on these expectations. Although our patient population and its response to treatment may vary considerably, its variation can still be measured. Depending on homogeneity of outcome and number of patients, it may take collection of data for a few months or a year before we decide that we understand the variability.

Table 2. MULTIPLE CUSTOMERS AND THEIR NEEDS IN A PAIN CASE

Customer	Possible needs
Patient	Less pain
	Maintenance of income
	Maintenance of job esteem
	Maintenance of avocational activities
	Cutting of individual health care cost
	Maintenance of family integrity
	Decreased worry about the future, diagnosis, and so on
Employer	Productive work from the employee
	Lower health insurance payment
	Lower out-of-pocket health payment
	Maintenance of work force morale, union relations
	Decreased paperwork
	Decreased risk of lawsuit, OSHA citation
	Clearly defined work restrictions
Insurer	Improved profitability of insurance
	Lower medical payments
	Quick disposition
	Rapid termination of case and permanency rating
	Quick, complete paperwork
Case manager	Maintenance of income
	Low case cost
	Predictable case cost
	Rapid termination of case and permanency rating
	Access to doctor
	Influence over referrals
	Quick, complete paperwork
Referring physician	Easy dismissal of a difficult or uninteresting case
	Validation of clinical judgment
	Reciprocal referral
	Control over other aspects of the patient
	Better outcome than the referrer could have achieved
	Maintenance of income and referrals
Therapy team	Professional and personal respect
	Complete information
	Easy access to physician
	Clear direction, yet room for independent judgment
	Appropriate reimbursement
	Recognition of special effort
Family, friends, co-workers, other insurers, and attorneys all have other needs	

Data collection is typically shied away from by nonuniversity types but is not all that hard. This approach does not require the randomized, double-blinded, Greek-alphabet-soup statistical approach. Just means and standard deviations of measures that you as a clinician think are relevant are all that is usually needed. Without an honest objective measure of our work, it is difficult to claim that we have had an impact at all on our patients. The cost in time and effort is minimal, and it probably pays for itself in staff morale, office efficiency, and new referrals. We have proposed elsewhere a few simple outcome measures that can be measured in worker rehabilitation programs.[3] Briefly, an office practice might divide patients into acute, subacute, and chronic presentation; keep track of their age, sex, job type, and previous surgery; and call them up after discharge to find out whether they returned to work within a week or two of discharge and whether they were still at work 6 months later.

The fourth step is to review the data in light of the "manufacturing" process that we use. Are some cases clear outliers? Outliers are not just the best half or best third of our cases but the cases that fall more than two standard deviations beyond our usual variation. Why did the outliers do so well or so poorly? Can we use this experience in other cases? Are there treatments or processes that we have learned of recently (from the literature, colleagues, the Booz Allen approach, or our own innovation) that might improve our outcome? Our goal is not to react to variation inherent in the system but to improve the system itself. We decide on modifications to try and what measures will help us to detect changes.

The fifth step is to treat another cycle of patients using the changes in our protocol of assessment of customer needs, change, measurement of outcome, etc. The Deming cycle continues with quarterly or annual changes that result in CQI.

CONCLUSIONS: THE EVOLUTION OF YOUR PRACTICE

Conclusion? We can't be done yet! The references haven't reached double digits yet. Where is the foolproof algorithm that we can mindlessly plug into our practice? How can we address the functional needs of our pain patients without facts? We need facts.

It is a prerequisite that the physician who manages people with chronic pain know the current literature. Most of us think we do, but for back pain alone, *Index Medicus* lists more than 100 review articles and 1000 titles in the past 3 years. How do we read all of this? Do we really include every proven treatment in our management of every patient? Or do we choose based on our personal skills, resources, and biases? When we do mimic a successful therapy, do we execute it correctly? What if we are the ones with the innovative ideas? In our practice lifetime, we will be most able to improve our patient's function if we are able to change our practice pattern with an element of sanity.

In this article we introduced a model for change. We had fun disguising it as a business technique, but the methods are most deeply rooted in the practice of medicine. First, the model requires that we strive to understand the patient's functional needs. We propose that this is best done by eliciting the information from the patient before attempting a diagnosis. This is just a different approach to history taking. Second, we warn ourselves not to be the cause of iatrogenic disability: "primum non nocere" in disguise. Finally, we suggest a critical and methodologic assessment of all of the factors in and out of our practice that may interfere with the functional outcome of our treatment. When we make changes in our practice, we take responsibility to measure whether they have improved outcome. Here, we are just taking the observation and scientific methodology we learned in medical school out into the field.

The management of disability is an inseparable part of the management of pain. Even if we cannot cure pain, we can almost always do something to improve disability. We can avoid a lot of the dissatisfaction with futile attempts to manage pain by instead working to manage the disability. It is crucial that we understand our patient's real goals, that we simplify the process of care, and that we collect data within our own practices to assess the effect of changes we make.

ACKNOWLEDGMENTS

The author thanks Roger Gerard of Novus Healthcare Corporation for his perspectives on quality assurance in health care and Brenda K. Vander Zanden for assistance in manuscript preparation.

References

1. Bigos SJ, Battie MC: Acute care to prevent back disability: Ten years of progress. Clin Orthop 221:121–130, 1987
2. Deming WE: Out of the Crisis. Cambridge, Massachusetts Institute of Technology, 1986
3. Haig AJ, Penha S: Worker rehabilitation programs—separating fact from fiction. West J Med 154:528–531, 1991
4. Healthcare Productivity Report: Patient-focused care at Bishop Clarkson Hospital scores improvements in patient satisfaction in a radical new design of the hospital workplace: A case study. 4:5, May 1991
5. McEachern JE, Makens PK, Buchanan ED, et al: Quality improvement: An imperative for medical care. J Occup Med 33:365–371, 1991
6. Nachemson A: Work for all, for those with low back pain as well. Clin Orthop 179:78–85, 1983
7. Neave HR: The Deming Dimension. Knoxville, SPC Press, 1990
8. Twemlow SW, Gabbard GO: Iatrogenic disease or doctor-patient collusion? Am Fam Physician 24:129–134, 1987

Address reprint requests to

Andrew J. Haig, MD
Center for Rehabilitation Services
130 Second Street
Neenah, WI 54956

DISABILITY PREVENTION AND MANAGEMENT

Michel Lacerte, MDCM, MSc, FRCPC

The office physician rarely finds a situation more difficult to deal with than the patient with chronic pain and disability. The number of such disability claims is taking alarming proportions.[1, 2, 7]

Medical schools traditionally rooted in the medical model are currently not responding to this societal crisis. Unable to provide a medical cure and ill equipped to deal with the combination of chronic pain and disability, the physician who perceives himself as the patient's advocate often feels justified in supporting the disability claim.

This article presents a clinical approach for the prevention, recognition, and management of disability associated with chronic pain. An attribution theory based approach is suggested to facilitate the process of determining contributing factors (attributes) to illness behaviors. A methodology to analyze and develop a rehabilitation plan favoring interventions that maximize residual abilities is presented. Principles of prevention and management of chronic pain and disability syndrome are provided.

BACKGROUND

The term *disability* causes a great degree of confusion because its definition is dependent on whether we are using it within a medical, legal, or administrative context. Criteria, definition, and determination of disability vary among jurisdictions, agencies, and professions. The absence of widely used uniform standards and methodology for evaluating disability further compounds this issue. For the purpose of this article, disability is defined as "any restriction or lack of ability to perform an activity in the manner or within the range considered normal for a human being.

From the University of Western Ontario, London, Ontario, Canada

PHYSICAL MEDICINE AND REHABILITATION CLINICS
OF NORTH AMERICA

Temporary, total, or partial disability for a specific occupation is a predictable and medically appropriate state secondary to a large number of injuries and illnesses. Strang[33] defines chronic pain and disability syndrome as follows:

1. Being out of work continually for a minimum of 6 months and reporting a subjective conviction of being disabled and entitled to monetary payments, whether received or not
2. Having subjective complaints that are out of proportion to the degree of actual objective impairments
3. Having important psychological features (confirmed by psychological testing and clinical examination, whether overt or covert and whether acknowledged or denied) that underlie and reflect the subjective complaints and influence the conviction of disability and dependence on disability payments
4. Having a decreased or absent motivation to recover actively and a negative attitude about returning to work
5. All features must be present for a minimum of 6 months and not be due to any other recognized discrete medical or psychiatric condition

If the acute medical model is used, the disability state should cease as the illness is managed or the injury is healed. The challenge arises when the disability state fails to vanish following the usual healing period and pain persists beyond a medically reasonable time frame.

When facing such a challenge, resorting to the clinical method is particularly important because it forces the clinician to proceed in a series of logical steps beginning with the collection of observational data. In the case of chronic pain and disability, observations of behaviors and functions are of primary importance.

Although each datum is interpreted in the Cartesian model in light of the known biologic facts of anatomy, physiology, and biochemistry, it is believed that psychological and social influences can also modulate individual perception of and response to disease (biopsychosocial model).[8, 34]

The synthesis of the data collected suggests a series of hypotheses that in turn are tested in light of further observations to formulate one or several working diagnoses making up a problem list. Each working diagnosis is continuously evaluated as medical interventions are made. The biopsychosocial model suggests that medical interventions may not be sufficient to manage the chronic pain and disability syndrome.[7]

To identify and measure potential psychological and social influences on illness behaviors, an attribution theory approach is suggested (Fig. 1.)

A two-stage model for diagnosing and selecting interventions to address pain and disability behaviors is proposed. The first stage of the model consists of the attribution or diagnostic stage. The clinician attempts to attribute cause(s) to observed or reported behavior(s). It is naive to believe that a specific behavior can be caused by only one attribute; however, the attribution process does provide a logical modus operandi. Analysis and planning (decision making) is the second stage of the model, during which possible biopsychosocial interventions are evaluated and selected.

Attributes can be divided into two major classes: internal and external.[32] Internal attributes include individual factors such as personality traits, moods, and interest. People who regard themselves as responsible for something that happens in their lives are making internal attribution. External attributes are environmental and outer factors, such as fate, luck, family, company, insurer,

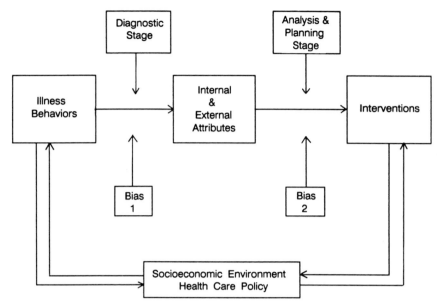

Figure 1. A model of biopsychosocial response to illness behavior.

and doctors, that are considered to be responsible for behaviors. The way in which people differ in their tendency to make either internal or external attributions is called *locus of control*. People who believe that they have control over their own destiny have an internal locus of control. Those who believe that their fate is under the control of other forces have an external locus of control.[30]

The following three rational factors underlying the attribution process must be understood.[32]

Distinctiveness. Distinctiveness is the extent to which an individual exhibits the same pattern of behavior in a variety of situations. The less distinctive the performance, the more likely the attribute is external (e.g., the individual reports being totally disabled for every imaginable task).

Consistency. Consistency is the extent to which the same behavior is exhibited over repetitions of the same situation. The greater the consistency, the more likely the attribute is internal (e.g., the back patient who exhibits the same range of motion at each office visit demonstrates internal consistency).

Consensus. Consensus refers to the extent to which other individuals exhibit similar behavior while performing the same tasks. The lower the consensus, the more likely the attribute is internal (e.g., the greater an individual performance deviates from standardized test norm, the more likely the attribution is internal).

It is critical that the physician consciously make internal and external attribution, or both, for a given illness behavior prior to the selection of intervention. A rehabilitation plan can then be developed to reduce or eliminate negative influences while maximizing positive influences on healthy behavior.

The physician must be aware that bias is usually introduced at both stages of the model because of their own values, beliefs, and training. The common statement that "it's another one of those compensation back cases" is an example of bias 1 found during the diagnostic stage. Another example of bias 1 is that, by training, the physician rightly attempts to eliminate possible organic causes (internal attributes) prior to exploring other causes (external attributes). Bias 2 may be introduced when funding for interventions is limited to the traditional medical remedies. In this situation, the treating physician has limited options and may resort to using ineffective but funded medical interventions. For example, an otherwise healthy individual unwilling to go back to work because of fear of losing both health and disability benefits will not be helped with more physical therapy (traditional) interventions. A benefit specialist must address this administrative issue.

DIAGNOSTIC STAGE

History

During history taking, the physician should make inquiries about multiple psychosocial factors that may contribute to illness behaviors.

Accident Factors

When basic identification data are collected, the patient should explain the reason for referral and the expectations from the consultation. The physician should pay particular attention to events surrounding the current claim of disability. Specific inquiry about personal losses and stresses that may have occurred prior to or around the time of the injury should be made. Recent work absences and vacation information can also be helpful. A detailed description of the accident and circumstances leading to a stressful incident or work absence is particularly important.

Medical Management Factors

Inquiry about how the injury was managed from the time of the accident to the present should be made. Particular attention should be paid to how the injury and disability have been explained and how they are understood by the patient. Information about interventions to date should then be obtained. Each intervention outcome, in terms of pain level and increased ability to function, should be recorded. This is particularly important because some interventions may, in fact, reinforce a sense of helplessness and disability. Feeling disabled is, by itself, disabling. Depression symptoms must be elicited, and a review of systems should be done to address all possible somatic complaints.

Pain Factors

To gain the necessary therapeutic trust of the patient, the physician would be wise to spend a lot of time with and to show genuine interest in the patient while taking the pain history. The use of a pain diagram and a pain rating scale facilitates this process.

Disability Factors

A functional activity screen provides information about activities of daily living, homemaking, avocational activities, lifestyle, and cognitive and interactive functions. During the interview, the patient should be asked to specify the cause of each limitation or perceived disability.

Claim Factors

Basic information about the disability claim, such as the claim number, date of accident, name of employer, name of third-party payer, whether the claim has been allowed or appealed, and whether payments have been received, should be documented. Inquiry should be made about previous disability claims and their courses and resolutions.

Employment Factors

Inquiries about employment-related factors provide valuable information about the socioeconomic environment of work. Psychosocial attributes related to job satisfaction and return-to-work barriers should be sought. Details should be obtained about the following:

Employment status at the time of injury and length of time at that job
The last day worked
Prior job changes and reasons for these
Current employment status and whether or not the employer is holding the preinjury job
Level of seniority
Union or professional-organization membership
Outstanding grievances or disciplinary issues
Job satisfaction, including items such as work atmosphere or the presence of monotonous and repetitive tasks
Attendance record over the past 5 years
Planned layoffs, expansions, or job changes
Employer and labor attitudes toward people with disabilities
Presence of a disability management program
The availability of modified work and time restrictions
Attempts at returning to work, including information about when, for how long, success, and factors contributing to failure

Family, Cultural, and Community Factors

Family, cultural, and community factors can often act as reinforcers of disability. Inquiry about family members or friends having had a similar disability and the outcome is helpful. Changes in family role, child-care arrangements, and so on are relevant.

Economic Factors

Information about the preaccident and current financial situation should be addressed. Delays or difficulties in obtaining disability benefits can represent major sources of stress. Inquiry about the relationship existing between patient and third-party payer is usually very insightful.

Legal Factors

The involvement of an attorney (why, for how long, and to what extent) can reveal important psychosocial attributes. For example, an attempt to return a patient back to work may be clinically indicated but may enter into direct conflict with the attorney's attempt to obtain a large settlement.

Physical Examination

In view of the relative absence of objective medical findings, attention should be paid to the functional abilities demonstrated by the patient during the interview. General appearance; handshake; stamina; pain behaviors; cognitive functions; mood; and lying, sitting, and standing tolerances should be noted. Gait, range of motion, and quality of body movements should be closely observed. The Waddell Nonorganic Physical Signs Test should become a routine part of the physical examination.[36]

At the completion of the history taking and physical examination, the physician is faced with identifying multiple potential attributes responsible for or modulating individual behaviors. Prior to coming up with a more definitive problem list, the physician may choose to make use of various assessment/screening tools. Table 1 represents a partial listing of some of the more commonly used tools.

ANALYSIS AND PLANNING STAGE

During the analysis and planning (decision-making) stage, attributes are analyzed in preparation of a rehabilitation plan. It is recommended that each attribute be reviewed in relation to the rational factors of the diagnostic stage (distinctiveness, consistency, and consensus) and the presence of bias factors.

The physician, cognizant of his or her own limitations to address some of these attributes, may choose to request the assistance of other disciplines (psychiatrist, psychologist, social worker, occupational therapist, and others).

Attributes can be gathered for analysis purpose in a structure called the Life Ability Box (LAB). The LAB (Fig. 2) facilitates the analysis of the possible interactions between different factors and attributes. The components of the LAB consist of medical disability, functional capacity, individual life demands, and psychosocial factors, all found within a socioeconomic environment. Internal attributes, associated with behavior and personality traits, are found among the individual psychosocial factors. The physician must be aware of environmental strengths, weakness, opportunities, and threats (external attributes) of the socioeconomic environment and how they could affect the other components.

To determine which attribute should be tackled first, it is advantageous to remember Maslow's hierarchy of needs[22] and the stages of adjustment as presented by Kubler-Ross[16] (i.e., denial, anger, bargaining, depression, and acceptance). A patient is very reluctant to participate if his physiologic (biologic) and safety needs are not first assured and depression not addressed.

Interventions derived from the LAB serve to bridge the gaps between the current disability state and the estimated maximal functional capacity. The physician must be prepared to deal with varying psychosocial needs that accompany the chronic pain and disability syndrome. The response to these needs would likely require interventions from a host of professionals in health, vocational rehabilitation counseling, psychology, social work, engineering, education, labor, insurance, and law. The interventions may be conducted in different environments such as hospitals, clinics, work sites, agencies, and home. Coordination of the implementation of the rehabilitation plan is time consuming but crucial.

Principles of Disability Prevention and Management

The elaboration of a prevention and management strategy to address the complex nature of chronic pain and disability syndrome should be based on a set of basic principles.

Prevention

Many prevention approaches reside with legislators, judges, third-party payers, employers, and physicians. Policy makers should reinforce that remaining an active member of society is preferable to receiving disability benefits or social assistance. For example, overcompensation of injured workers undermines the interest to return to work, especially if the employment conditions are perceived as less than satisfactory. The introduction of the Americans with Disabilities Act is one step in the right direction and should remove some of the employers' barriers.

By using the biopsychosocial model, the legal system can be viewed as an external attribute for adopting a disabled role. Ongoing litigation or compensation disputes may counteract what the rehabilitation process is attempting to accomplish. Early mediation and arbitration would be beneficial. On the other hand, attorneys can relieve the client from a lot of stress by ensuring that health and rehabilitation benefits funding is obtained. The patient can then concentrate all his or her energy on the restoration and adjustment process rather than fighting eligibility and entitlement matters with a third party.

Employers should be guided in how to provide a safe and pleasant work environment. In addition, they should be supported by the community in their effort to accommodate people with disabilities.

The physician must adopt the biopsychosocial model and spend more time counseling his patient through the stages of adjustment. Focus towards residual abilities should be maintained. The physician must provide an optimistic outlook. Reassuring his patient that no serious or fatal disease was found and that the prognosis is very good is crucial.[7]

Early Detection and Intervention

It is of the utmost importance to recognize as quickly as possible the signs of adoption of a sick role. Spending time educating the patient about the nature of chronic pain and the difference between hurt and harm is, indeed, time well spent.

Careful case management and coordination of consultations are essential. Where indicated, psychiatric consultation and treatment should be initiated as early as possible. Early referral to an interdisciplinary pain management program is highly recommended. The key characteristic of a good program is the presence of a group of professionals committed to and genuinely interested in restoring functional ability in individuals with chronic pain. (See article by Stanton later in this issue.)

Partnership

The patient is the most important partner in the development of the rehabilitation plan. It is essential that the individual participate, with the assistance of the treating physician and rehabilitation counselor, in setting up realistic rehabili-

Table 1. ATTRIBUTE IDENTIFICATION USING SCREENING TOOLS

Attributes	Screening Tools	Relevant Aspects
Internal Personality factors	Millon Behavior Health Inventory,[13] Eysenck Personality Questionnaire,[9] MMPI[6]	Emotions, frustration tolerance, self-esteem, achievement motivation, sense of autonomy, interest, satisfaction, commitment, psychiatric illness, personality disorders
Pain and illness experience	McGill Pain Questionnaire,[23, 24] Modified Somatic Perception Questionnaire,[20] Sickness Impact Profile,[3] Millon Visual Analog,[26] Linear Pain Scale,[15] Pain Drawing[28]	Patterns of intensity, quality changes, precipitating factors, relieving factors, reactive thoughts or feelings, beliefs about pain, health and illness attitude, future expectations
Pain context	McGill Pain Questionnaire,[23, 24] Psychosocial Pain Inventory[14]	Multiple conditions throughout life, chronic pain in family history, secondary gains, stressful events, pain behavior
Mood (depression)	Beck Depression Inventory,[2] Modified Zung Depression Inventory,[21, 41] Modified Somatic Perception Questionnaire[20]	Depression, anxiety, hopelessness
Coping skills and defense mechanisms	Lazarus and Folkman Ways of Coping Questionnaire,[12] Vanderbilt Pain Management Inventory,[5] Coping Strategies Questionnaire[29]	Stress management and regulating emotions, defense mechanisms: denial, repression, fantasy, projection, sublimation, escape, minimizing

Cognitive functions	WAIS-R[39]	Intelligence, concentration, attention, reasoning (verbal and spatial), short- and long-term memory, judgment and comprehension of social conventions
External		
Interpersonal relationships at the workplace	Work APGAR[4]	Job satisfaction
Family situation	Family interview, Family APGAR[31]	Stability and harmony of family, stress and effects of illness and pain in other family members
Social situation	Schema Assessment Inventory[18]	Quality and range of relationships, community support, litigation, compensation
Locus of control	Multidimensional Health Locus of Control Scale,[37, 38] Pain Related Control Scale,[11] Pain Related Self Statements scale[11]	Perception of self as effective agent versus a sense of helplessness, sense of others being in control
Functional activity	Waddell Disability Index,[35] Oswestry LBP Disability Questionnaire,[10] Functional Assessment Screen Questionnaire,[25] Dallas Low Back Pain Questionnaire[19]	Type, specific description, secondary gains, attitudes related to the pain behaviors, reinforcing contingencies
Medication use	Pain rating and medication diary	Type, frequency, pain relief, side effects, attitudes toward medication use, fears about addiction

19

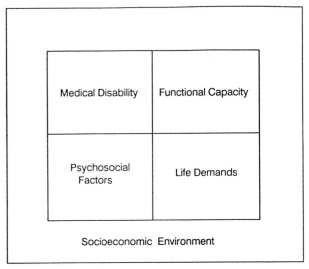

Figure 2. The Life Ability Box.

tation goals, objectives, and timetables. The support of family, employer, attorney, and others is necessary for the successful outcome of the rehabilitation plan.

Goal-Oriented Rehabilitation Plan

The rehabilitation plan must have clearly delineated goals, objectives, responsibilities, and timetables. All the parties must understand their roles and responsibilities in the process. The rehabilitation plan must be flexible and allow for change in accordance with the circumstances.

Independence of Medical Decision Making from Entitlement

The physician must be aware of his patient's legal and administrative circumstances but should avoid getting pulled into the determination of entitlement to benefits or services. The physician should refuse to be forced into collusion over disability claim entitlement issues. The physician's role is to determine whether there are medical reasons why an individual should not engage in doing certain activities (occupational fitness determination). The physician should be careful not to take over from the claim adjudicator the administrative decision about eligibility or entitlement. It is appropriate for a physician to say that an individual is permanently totally disabled for doing the essential tasks of his preinjury occupation. It is inappropriate for the physician to say that an individual is eligible and entitled for a long-term disability pension, which is a nonmedical administrative function.[17]

Respect and Dignity

Clinicians must act at all times within the code of ethics and respect the patient's right to make the wrong decision (empowerment). The physician should advise the patient about the potential consequences of his decisions.

Quality Assurances

Active treatment programs focusing on improving functional capacity (be it at home or at the workplace) are favored over passive approaches such as bed rest, massage, and diathermy, which are sick role reinforcers.

The clinician should critically appraise the literature when planning interventions, especially when they are new or unfamiliar to him.

Clinicians must strive to provide high-quality services to each patient. This can be achieved by monitoring and evaluating services delivered.

Case Study

John is a 51-year-old laborer at a tire manufacturing plant who claims having sustained, 4 months ago, a compensable low back injury while attempting to pull upright a loaded dolly that had fallen.

He sought immediate medical attention from his family physician, Dr. Smith, who attempted to follow, as closely as possible, the Critical Path for the Management of Spinal Disorders.[27] Dr. Smith provided John with much reassurance about the benign nature of his condition in addition to prescribing nonsteroidal anti-inflammatory drugs, analgesics, spasmolytics, and an active physical therapy program.

After 6 weeks of active physical therapy, John reported very little improvement in pain and functional activity levels. At 7 weeks, John had a consultation with a back specialist. The diagnosis of a mechanical low back pain was confirmed, and further reassurance as to the benign nature of his condition was given.

The specialist's recommendation was to intensify rehabilitation efforts, using the work site as a training ground (on-site transitional work return program). Furthermore, an occupational therapist and ergonomist should ensure that modified work is within prescribed medical restrictions. The disturbed sleeping pattern and self-report of depression were a source of concern.

Every 2 weeks, Dr. Smith monitored John's symptoms of pain and reports of disability, using a pain diagram, pain scale, and a functional index. Through this process, trust between the two was built. Dr. Smith counseled John during adjustment stages and was a constant source of optimism. Despite these efforts, the clinical records pointed toward chronicity.

At 3 months, while reviewing the model of biopsychosocial response to illness behavior, Dr. Smith noted a bias towards organicity. The psychosocial aspects of pain and disability (attributes) needed further exploration. Potential psychosocial barriers to recovery were exposed during the follow-up visit.

Accident Factors. The accident occurred on a Monday morning immediately after a 1-week vacation. John was working in an unfamiliar area of the plant managed by a new supervisor who is half his age. John did not particularly like working with the dolly.

Medical Management Factors. A review of John's past medical history revealed that 10 years ago, he sustained a work-related back injury that necessitated 6 months off work. Dr. Smith was aware of John's history of alcohol and substance abuse.

John expressed fear that something was being missed, despite reassurance by both Dr. Smith and the specialist. This belief had been reinforced by a physical therapist who had told him that he had a "disc problem." After being told this, John's attendance in physical therapy dropped below 60%. He stated that the exercises were making him worse. No one, to date, has explained to John the differences between hurt versus harm or provided back education.

John admitted having tried his brother's oxycodone tablets and reported that they were the only thing that significantly relieved his pain.

Pain Factors. On the pain rating scale, John consistently rated his pain at 9 on a scale of 0 to 10. Over the past month, John reported spreading of the pain over his entire back and lower extremities. He insisted that this feeling was real and not "in his head."

Disability Factors. John is convinced that he is totally disabled: "I can't do anything for any length of time. My wife has to do everything."

He reported that some mornings he cannot even get out of bed to go to therapy. He particularly misses his usual avocational interests, such as playing golf and gardening. John claims that returning to his old job would be impossible. He attributed his current condition to "bad luck" and negligence by his employer (external locus of control and attribution).

Claim Factors. John feels entitled to workers' compensation benefits. He is very upset that, after he has worked hard for the past 15 years, his employer is appealing the claim.

His rehabilitation is currently covered by his sick-and-accident-benefits insurance; however, his claim adjudicator has recently threatened to cut his benefits if he continued to demonstrate poor attendance.

Employment Factors. John has an eighth-grade education and limited English reading and writing skills. John likes to work alone and has no friends at work. Since the accident, no return-to-work attempts have been made, nor has there been communication with the employer.

John stated that the employer has no modified work and would not take him back unless he is 100%. John also stated that the employer is currently considering having massive layoffs or relocating to Mexico.

Family, Cultural, and Community Factors. John stated that many of his friends at the Mediterranean Café have permanent disability benefits and are in much better shape than he is. His younger brother has been on long-term disability for the past 7 years for the same problem. Consequently, John feels entitled to compensation and that he is "just too old to return to this type of work anyway."

John reported being quite frustrated with his new family role. He admitted being short-tempered with his wife and adult children. His marital situation, problematic prior to his accident, has since greatly deteriorated. He reported not having had sex since the accident.

Economic Factors. Prior to his accident, John was barely making ends meet, particularly since his wife had been laid off 6 months earlier. His home mortgage and car payments have just about eaten up his savings. John does not want to end up on welfare. He is particularly concerned with not being able to pay for his daughter's wedding in 2 months. He is not receiving any income and feels totally helpless.

Legal Factors. John met twice with an attorney, who assured him that there would be no cost unless they win. He stated that John had a good claim but it may take time before any money is received. John said that the attorney had other clients who benefited from chiropractic adjustment, mud baths, and massage therapy.

On physical examination, Dr. Smith noted minimal abnormalities in John's gait, back range of motion, and quality of movement. He also noted the presence of Waddell's nonorganic physical signs.

To complete his assessment, Dr. Smith used a number of assessment and screening tools, including the modified Zung depression inventory, the Multidimensional Health Locus of Control Scale, and the Oswestry Low Back Pain Questionnaire.

Dr. Smith developed a problem list made up of potential internal and external attributes contributing to John's illness behavior. Effective utilization of the LAB required Dr. Smith to have information relative to current functional capacity. A functional capacity evaluation was therefore needed to assess whether John was physically capable to perform the essential tasks of his job. It was also realized that life-demands information relative to his preaccident occupation (e.g., essential tasks description) was also missing. Furthermore, the employer had never directly been asked to provide clarification about its disability management policies.

Despite the missing information, Dr. Smith recognized early signs of chronic pain and disability syndrome. In view of the complexity of the situation, he chose to make a referral to an interdisciplinary ability restoration outpatient program as discussed in the article by Stanton, with the rehabilitation goal to provide better pain coping skills rather than elimination of the pain. Objectives of the program would be to manage each internal and external attribute.

After having made the referral, John informed Dr. Smith that his insurance company does not provide funding for such a program but would fund massage therapy. Dr. Smith was distressed because his best medical recommendations were not being funded or carried out. Dr. Smith gradually decreased his involvement as John was being consumed by the litigation process.

Despite the unsatisfactory ending to this case study, there are several lessons to be learned. First, physicians must reject the traditional medical model in favor of the biopsychosocial approach to include psychosocial factors as attributes of illness behaviors. Second, the LAB should be used to analyze attributes and plan appropriate interventions. Finally, the use of principles of disability prevention and management help in dealing with the complex nature of chronic pain and disability syndrome.

CONCLUSION

People who have sustained an injury associated with a disability are often unprepared to deal with or adjust to its physical, psychological, and socioeconomic consequences.

To address this diagnostic challenge and to recognize the early signs of the syndrome, the physician must adopt the biopsychosocial and rehabilitation models.

The management of chronic pain and disability syndrome is daunting for most office physicians and requires time, knowledge, dedication, and a great deal of patience. If the office physician does not believe that he can effectively manage the onerous task of managing a team in addition to providing his own interventions, he should make sure not to reinforce the sick role. This physician should become familiar with and use the principles of disability prevention and management:

prevention
early detection and interventions
partnership

goal-oriented rehabilitation plan
independence of medical decision making from entitlement
respect and dignity
quality assurance

References

1. Berkowitz M: Disability expenditures, 1970–1982. Report No. 6, National Institute of Handicapped Research, Project No. 133AH3005. Bureau of Economic Research, Rutgers University, 1985
2. Beck AT, Ward CH, Mendelson M, et al: An inventory for measuring depression. Arch Gen Psychiatry 4:561–571, 1961
3. Bergner M, Bobbitt RA, Carter WB, et al: The Sickness Impact Profile: Development and final revision of a health status measure. Med Care 19:787–805, 1981
4. Bigos SJ, Battie MC, Spengler DM, et al: A prospective study of work perceptions and psychosocial factors affecting the report of back injury. Spine 16:1–6, 1991
5. Brown GK, Nicassio PM: Development of a questionnaire for the assessment of active and passive coping strategies in chronic pain patients. Pain 31:53–65, 1987
6. Dahlstrom WG, Welsh GS: An MMPI Handbook. Minneapolis, University of Minnesota Press, 1960
7. Deyo RA, Cherkin D, Conrad D, et al: Cost, controversy, crisis: Low back pain and the health of the public. Annu Rev Public Health 12:141–156, 1991
8. Engel GL: The need for a new medical model: A challenge for biomedicine. Science 196:129–136, 1977
9. Eysenck HJ, Eysenck SBG: Manual of the Eysenck Personality Questionnaire. Seven Oaks, Kent Hodden & Stoughton, 1975
10. Fairbank JL, Cooper J, Davies JB, et al: The Oswestry low back pain questionnaire. Physiotherapy 66:271, 1980
11. Flor H, Turk DC: Rheumatoid arthritis and back pain: Predicting pain and disability from cognitive variables. J Behav Med 11:251–265, 1988
12. Folkman S, Lazarus RS: If it changes it must be a process: A study of emotion and coping during three stages of a college examination. J Pers Soc Psychol 48:150–170, 1985
13. Gatchel R, Mayer T, Capra P, et al: Millon Behavioral Health Inventory: Its utility in predicting physical function in patients with low back pain. Arch Phys Med Rehabil 67:878–882, 1986
14. Heaton RK, Getto CJ, Lehman RAW, et al: A standardized evaluation of psychosocial factors in low back pain. Pain 12:165–174, 1982
15. Huskisson EC: Measurement of pain. Lancet 2:1127, 1974
16. Kubler-Ross E: On Death and Dying. New York, Macmillan, 1985
17. Lacerte M, Wright G: Return to work determination. Physical Medicine & Rehabilitation: State of the Art Reviews 6:283–302, 1991
18. Lacroix JM: Illness schemata: Emerging methodological and empirical issues. Canadian Psychology 28:225, 1987
19. Lawlis GF, Cuencas R, Selby D, et al: The development of a Dallas pain questionnaire: An assessment of the impact of spinal pain on behavior. Spine 14:511, 1989
20. Main CJ: The Modified Somatic Perception Questionnaire. J Psychosom Res 27:503–514, 1983
21. Main CJ, Waddell G: The detection of psychological abnormality in chronic low back pain patients using four simple scales. Current Concepts in Pain 2:10–15, 1984
22. Maslow A: Motivation and Personality. New York, Harper & Row, 1954
23. Melzack R: The McGill Pain Questionnaire: Major properties and scoring methods. Pain 1:277–299, 1975
24. Melzack R: The short-form McGill Pain Questionnaire. Pain 30:191–197, 1987
25. Millard RW: The functional assessment screening questionnaire: Application for evaluating pain-related disability. Arch Phys Med Rehabil 70:303–307, 1989

26. Millon R, Wall W, Nilsen K, et al: Assessment of the progress of the back pain patient. Spine 7:204, 1982
27. Québec Task Force on Spinal Disorders: Scientific approach to the assessment and management of activity-related spinal disorders: A monograph for clinicians. Spine 12(suppl 7), 1987
28. Ransford AO, Douglas C, Mooney V: The pain drawing as an aid to the psychologic evaluation of patients with low back pain. Spine 1:127, 1976
29. Rosenstiel AK, Keefe FJ: The use of coping strategies in chronic low back pain patients: Relationship to patient characteristics and current adjustments. Pain 17:33–34, 1983
30. Scarpello VG, Ledvinka J: Personnel/Human Resource Management: Environments and Functions. Boston, PWS-Kent, 1988, pp 32–33
31. Smilkstein G: The family APGAR: A proposal for family function test and its use by physicians. J Fam Pract 6:1231–1235, 1978
32. Steers RM, Porter LW: Motivation and Work Behavior, ed 4. New York, McGraw-Hill, 1987, p 419
33. Strang JP: The chronic disability syndrome. In Aronoff GM (ed): Evaluation and Treatment of Chronic Pain. Baltimore, Urban & Schwarzenberg, 1985, pp 603–623
34. Waddell G: A clinical model for the treatment of low-back pain. Spine 12:632–644, 1987
35. Waddell G, Main CJ, Morris EW, et al: Chronic low back pain, psychologic distress and illness behavior. Spine 9:209–213, 1984
36. Waddell G, McColloch JA, Kummel ED, et al: Nonorganic physical signs in low back pain. Spine 5:117–125, 1980
37. Wallston KA, Wallston BS: Health locus of control scales. In Lefcourt HM (ed): Research with the Locus of Control Construct, vol 1. New York, Academic Press, 1981, pp 189–243
38. Wallston KA, Wallston BS, DeVillis R: Development of the Multidimensional Health Locus of Control (MHLC) scales. Health Education Monographs 6:160–170, 1978
39. Wechsler D: WAIS-R Manual: Wechsler Adult Intelligence Scale–Revised. San Antonio, Psychological Corporation, 1981
40. World Health Organization: International Classification of Impairments, Disabilities, and Handicaps. Geneva, World Health Organization, 1980
41. Zung WWK: A self-rated depression scale. Arch Gen Psychiatr 32:63, 1965

Address reprint requests to

Dr. Michel Lacerte
801 Commissioners Road East
London, Ontario 56C 5J1, Canada

THE PROBLEM PATIENT WITH PAIN

From Myth to Mayhem

Daniel V. Voiss, MS, MD

The title of this issue, *Office Management of Pain,* directs our attention to one of the major difficulties in all areas of current medical practice: focus on the symptom instead of on the patient. In this article, I share with you my observations, analysis, and comments regarding this problem and the risks to patients when we become preoccupied with the suppression of symptoms without understanding the patient. Whether a symptom or a verbal complaint is fashionable or acceptable medically determines, to a large extent, whether it is presented by the patient. Problem Patients with Pain are very serious about their complaints, and they do not wish to be dismissed, rejected, or ridiculed. They present symptoms that suggest a legitimate medical disorder, and the more that they are examined, the more specific and fine-tuned their complaints become.[58, 59, 64] The symptoms of these patients are real, but their hypothesis as to the cause of the complaints, which they verbalize, is inaccurate and invalid. This faulty clinical hypothesis is the sine qua non of the Problem Patient with Pain. Therefore, it is not the "pain" that needs to be managed but the patient who needs to be understood so that we can assist him or her in "managing" himself or herself; this is a disorder of adaptation.

"Pain," as a verbal and nonverbal complaint, is probably the most frequent symptom that brings a patient to medical attention. Any part of the body may be engaged: chest, abdomen, head, neck, back, and extremities. Sensory and motor complaints often include numbness, tingling, dizziness, weakness, and collapsing. These types of complaints are present in every area of medical practice: primary care, physiatry, neurology, medicine, orthopedics, and, last but not least, psychiatry.

Understanding the person of the patient is the cornerstone of appropriate, effective intervention, and this is particularly true for Problem Patients with Pain.

From ACCESS Consulting Systems Incorporated, Portland, Oregon

PHYSICAL MEDICINE AND REHABILITATION CLINICS
OF NORTH AMERICA

VOLUME 4 • NUMBER 1 • FEBRUARY 1993

When, as physicians, we focus our attention on symptoms, to the relative exclu-sion of understanding the contextual situation of our patients, who they are and their mental, emotional, and personal life situation, we practically guarantee the development of a Problem Patient with Pain. If we focus our attention upon understanding the body part and neglect the person of the patient, we relegate the patient to the status of a physiologic preparation, a laboratory animal. This neglect of the person may be appropriate for basic-science researchers but not for the practicing clinical physician.

It is obviously important to perform those clinical and laboratory studies indicated by particular symptoms or verbal complaints, but these tests should follow, not precede, the understanding of the individual who brings these com-munications of dysfunction to us for clarification, support, and assistance. Chronic pain symptoms are often communications of adaptive difficulties, pre-cipitated either by organic pathology or by adaptively initiated mental processes. It is well established that adaptively initiated brain activity and images provoke cortical neuronal group function that may elicit somatosensory, somatomotor, and autonomic responsiveness.[1, 12, 14, 16, 54] Unless we know something about the adapting organism, the person whom we have undertaken to assist, we are susceptible to misinterpreting and therefore misunderstanding their complaints. Comprehensive understanding of the patient is usually available only through a detailed individual history or, in some cases, medical records and other collateral sources. Obtaining this history is often easier advised than accomplished, partic-ularly when working with a Problem Patient with Pain, because the bodily symptoms represent a psychological defense against painful ideas, images, and affects. Consequently, the history that we are able to elicit may not be the history that we need to make an accurate diagnosis. These patients are attempting to adapt to current circumstances by remaining unaware of the real issues that promote their seeking medical involvement, or if aware, unable or unwilling to communicate them.

There are two common but understandable explanations for this situation: first, the patients may be aware of aspects of their adaptive style, their personal life, that they do not wish to divulge because they are ashamed or embarrassed or fear criticism and hostility from the physician or others.

An example of this type of situation is provided by a 38-year-old woman who was referred for psychiatric, psychological, and neurologic evaluation because of complaints of pain in her dominant left upper extremity that followed a minor bump to her left shoulder that resulted in no obvious clinical findings. She presented with complaints of pain, numbness, tingling, and weakness. She had observable but minimal atrophy of the left upper extremity and forearm. Electro-myography and nerve conduction studies were bilaterally normal, except for absent distal latencies of the left superficial radial nerve. Symptoms eventually expanded to include the right arm and also included cooling and complaints of color changes in both hands. Numerous diagnoses were considered, including carpal tunnel syndrome, radial nerve entrapment, deQuervain's tenosynovitis, reflex sympathetic dystrophy, impingement syndrome of the left shoulder, and even somatoform pain disorder. There was no personal information about this individual in any of the records, all of which were reviewed. It was as though personal information was either taboo or irrelevant. In effect, it appeared that the patient and physicians were unwittingly colluding in an effort to not make a diagnosis.[63] This young woman's complaints continued, intensified, and ex-panded for more than a year, during which she was paid by her employer and spent most of her time visiting physicians. Each consultant provided a new perspective, additional studies, a new diagnosis, and elicited new symptoms. An

MRI suggested a cervical disc protrusion at C6–7, and surgery was suggested; however, it would have been unreasonable and irresponsible in view of the repeatedly normal electric studies and absence of any significant clinical findings.[7, 8, 20, 28, 39, 41] The personal history of this woman, obtained during an audiotaped, transcribed clinical interview, revealed a chaotic, inconsistent, abusive, and disorganized personal development, which continued into adulthood. A detailed review of past medical care, including past and current medications, disclosed prior use of disulfiram ". . . years ago." The subsequent history revealed numerous arrests for driving while intoxicated and multiple job changes. Characteristic of chronic alcoholics, the patient denied drinking at this time, ". . . except an occasional beer"; however, neuromuscular pathology from alcoholism is very common and therefore needed to be assessed.[35, 36, 38, 42, 45] The peroneal and sural, in addition to the median and ulnar, nerves were then evaluated, using a nerve action potential assessment with current perception threshold technique. This has been reported as a useful test and independently assesses all three populations of nerve fibers. Furthermore, peripheral neuropathy generally appears earliest in the longest nerves.[9, 33, 40, 64]

Preliminary and computerized analysis of the data revealed values diagnostic of a diffuse peripheral polyneuropathy. All of this woman's complaints and the findings of mild muscle atrophy would be most reasonably explained on the basis of an undiagnosed diffuse polyneuropathy.[12, 13, 36] Laboratory studies ruled out diabetes, and the most likely diagnosis, under the circumstances, was alcoholic polyneuropathy, a condition more common than most of us probably care to recognize. This woman did not have a work-related injury to her nervous system, and nothing can be done for her unless she stops drinking. Surgery would have been harmful to the patient because it would have fixed her identification as a Problem Patient with Pain.

The second type of situation is one in which the Problem Patient with Pain is actually unaware of any of those factors that precipitate the focus of attention on the neuromusculoskeletal or other systems. Complaints of pain and other symptoms are unconsciously dissociated from the adaptively initiated, image-driven ideational and affective content that gives rise to them. The patient presents with a fixed belief with respect to the cause of the problem: cancer, minor injury, or other—under the circumstances—unlikely causative event. They cannot be dissuaded from their conviction as they travel an ever-expanding, eventually self-destructive journey through the health care system. If this odyssey is aided and abetted by attorneys and/or doctors, the likelihood of appropriately assisting the patient medically becomes increasingly remote because the Problem Patient with Pain has an advocate for his or her misperceptions and misunderstanding.[30, 31]

These Problem Patients with Pain present with what are most accurately described as somatic delusions. Such patients and the response they evoke in physicians have been comprehensively described in a number of classic articles. These are the patients whom responsible physicians and office staff usually learn to hate[2, 6, 26, 27, 53, 65]; however, such patients frequently are able to locate a physician who may unwittingly act as the facilitator of their self-destructive efforts.[37, 63]

An example of this type of situation is that of a 29-year-old woman who was referred for a comprehensive diagnostic assessment after pain in her upper extremities failed to improve subsequent to the following procedures: a carpal tunnel release, bilateral ulnar and radial nerve transpositions, and repeated stellate ganglion blocks. The surgeon who offered and provided these at-best-questionable procedures knew nothing about the life context of his Problem

Patient with Pain. Direct discussions with him elicited an opinion that personal information was irrelevant in view of this woman's continuing verbal complaints. The patient had recently moved to his area from another city. Two years prior to being seen by this surgeon and 3 years prior to being seen by us, she had bumped her right hand on a stove when she slipped and fell at work. She had a contusion and was evaluated, treated conservatively and appropriately, and released to return to work. Subsequently, she began to complain of spreading pain in the right and then the left upper extremities. She sought consultation and was seen by an orthopedist, a neurosurgeon, a neurologist, a physiatrist, two hand surgeons, and a vascular surgeon. At one point, a consulting hand surgeon had recommended psychiatric referral, but the patient declined and was supported in this refusal by the person handling her workers' compensation claim. She had been evaluated through multiple electric studies, including measurement of conduction velocities, electromyography, somatosensory-evoked potentials, and laser Doppler vascular studies, as well as numerous radiographs, MRIs, and bone scans, all of which were normal. Her complaints continued. Various diagnoses were offered: carpal tunnel syndrome, radial and ulnar nerve entrapment, thoracic outlet syndrome, reflex sympathetic dystrophy, and fibromyalgia. The emotional or adaptive difficulties of this particular patient were essentially unnoticed by the various consulting physicians, except by the surgeon who recommended psychiatric consultation. Those who did note something of an emotional nature with regard to ongoing complaints automatically attributed these emotional difficulties to the described injury; they confused cause and effect, thereby unwittingly colluding with the patient. This patient had no objective indications of neuromusculoskeletal pathology, and all of the physicians involved prior to her move to a new community had recommended against surgical intervention. If there was no objective evidence of injury, how could it cause her emotional problems? Major disruption in adaptive functioning, that is, emotional troubles, were attributed by the patient to a relatively minor event for which there was no clinical evidence of any pathology other than a short-term soft tissue injury. This patient's intransigent position with regard to her adaptive failures and their cause is totally consistent with the psychiatric diagnosis of a somatic delusion. To understand what this individual is presenting, we need to know more about her. We cannot "manage" her verbal complaints unless we are informed about the personal or adaptive context in which the incident occurred and the factors that cause her complaints to continue.

At the time this patient was seen for comprehensive evaluation by us, she described an ideal marital and family life; however, collateral information revealed that at the time of the incident that preceded her development as a Problem Patient with Pain, her husband had just abandoned her and their children for another woman. She was forced to go to work for the first time in her life. Shortly, thereafter, she was injured and embarked on her journey through many physicians' offices, metaphorically seeking help for her "pain" as she insisted on her continuing helplessness. Certainly, she was injured, but the real injury was not that which she identified, a minor soft tissue injury. The injury incident became the rationalization that allowed this Problem Patient with Pain to go from doctor to doctor, displaying her "hurt" and asking for help while repressing her feelings in regard to her predicament with her husband, by whom she had indeed been "injured." The real problem was not the hand. The patient could not allow herself conscious awareness of her painful and enraging loss. Because the problem was not a nerve injury, repeated electrodiagnostic and other procedures could not elucidate a cause for her complaints any more than the subsequent iatrogenically mutilating surgeries could cure them. Those procedures served to reinforce her somatic delusion and her role as a Problem Patient with Pain. When this patient moved to another city and took up residence with her husband's family, her complaints continued and she underwent the described surgical procedures. Nevertheless, her complaints continued unabated, and even more surgery was recommended. Through the continuing metaphoric display of how her husband had injured her, she was able to get him home, keep him home, and keep him under control. This individual appeared to have no conscious awareness of what she was doing and how she was doing it. The surgical treatment she received can best be described as "psychosurgery" because it enhanced her unconscious adaptive efforts, which were mental and not due to physical injury. She will demand, through her complaints, continuing surgical procedures to maintain her adaptation as a Problem Patient with Pain. The health care system is inundated with patients like the aforementioned two.

Ochoa has commented elsewhere in this issue, as well as in other articles, on the mythology of reflex sympathetic dystrophy.[46–48] The history of medicine and medical practice is a history of mythology.* Despite the tremendous proliferation of technical instruments for the establishment of "scientific diagnoses," the mythology continues.

For instance, in more than 600 Problem Patients with Pain in whom we have conducted comprehensive orthopedic, neurologic, and psychiatric–psychological evaluations over the past 10 years, less than 10% have demonstrated objective evidence of neuromusculoskeletal pathology. In those 10%, the anatomic and pathologic diagnoses could not account for the extent of disability with which the individual presented. This finding is consistent with studies on Problem Patients with Pain.[32, 63] Many of our patients were evaluated in conjunction with the staff of the Neuromuscular Unit, under Ochoa's supervision. Neurologic assessment consisted of detailed clinical evaluation, electromyography, nerve conduction measurements, somatosensory-evoked potentials, quantitative somatosensory thermotesting, laser Doppler, thermography, single-fiber nerve recordings, and, in some cases, nerve biopsy and electron microscopy. All the patients evaluated conjointly were seen for audiotaped, transcribed psychiatric interviews and administered a battery of psychological tests, which always included the Minnesota Multiphasic Personality Inventory (MMPI) and a Rorschach Ink Blot Test, scored by the Exner method. The MMPI and the Rorschach were computer analyzed, and narrative reports were generated from that data. Significant developmental, psychological, and adaptive difficulties were explicitly revealed in all individuals who were identified neurologically and by history as Problem Patients with Pain, that is, individuals in whom there were essentially no objective findings and had a continuing course of involvement with the health care system. They had evidence of absence of relevant organic neurologic dysfunction. The two major psychiatric diagnostic categories were depression, often associated with loss of a specific important person, and psychosis. Complaints of pain served a major adaptive function for these individuals and, in some cases, clearly assisted the patient in avoiding suicide or full-blown psychological disorganization.

As physicians, we need to think about the Problem Patient with Pain as an individual who is making a statement through which they are communicating about a feared or impending adaptive failure. Certainly, patients can present with both peripherally initiated organic pain complaints and adaptive failures at the same time. This can lead to overelaboration of an injury or some other event, which may be focused on the peripheral neuromusculoskeletal system by both

* References 4, 5, 21, 55, 57–59, and 61.

patients and physicians. These patients can also become Problem Patients with Pain; however, as a rule, when an accurate diagnosis is made and effective treatment initiated, this type of patient usually reverts to appropriate, reasonable, and adaptive interactions with physicians and staff.

In the preceding observations and comments, our attention has been directed to the adaptive aspects of the complaints with which our Problem Patients with Pain have presented. Adaptation is a function of the central nervous system—specifically, the brain. The brain is the organ of adaptation; "We are our brains."[49] The Cartesian dichotomy with which medicine and medical science have been encumbered since recorded history—that the mind and the body are separate—is the mythologic foundation on which most medical practice has come to rely. This is the mythology which has significantly contributed to the fractionation of patient care and the proclivity for "managing" patients as physiologic preparations rather than analyzing symptoms as possible metaphoric expressions of dysfunction of the total patient. That is, symptoms are often taken out of context. The mind and the brain are inseparable. The mind is what the brain does, and the body and the brain are inseparable; therefore, the body is as much mind as the brain.

Brain development, our development as individuals, depends on the presence of adequate genetic programming for the evolution of the basic synaptic organization or structure of the brain, referred to by Edelman as the "primary repertoire."[17] Genetically determined organization provides the framework from which subsequent development moves; however, the primary determinant of the adaptive aspects of brain development is experience, or the environmental input, that is, early human development. Experientially derived synaptic organization results in the development of the "secondary repertoire."[18] Any casual observer of animals or humans knows that an active, modulated, enriched, and protected developmental environment increases the individual's mental capacities and adaptive resources. Synaptic interactions and the development of selective neuronal groups, the essential cortical processing units, are primarily dependent on the developmental history of the brain, that is, the developmental history of the individual.[12–14, 16] Adaptively initiated memories and associated images may give rise to activity in neuronal groups. The areas activated determine the response of the individual. Because the brain is connected, activation in one area may have widespread consequences and involve other areas, and it is this process which provokes symptom spreading. Man's adaptation occurs through and within his brain. As Edelman[15] notes in his thesis on consciousness, man is the only animal capable of modeling the world free of the present. Memory can bring the past dramatically into the present and, at the same time, precipitate a host of sensory and physiologic experiences, usually in response to imagery—primarily, if not exclusively, a thought modality of the right brain. All sensory experiences, including pain, have memory correlates that may be evoked without requiring specific external stimuli.[1, 49] In the absence of a functioning, conscious organ of adaptation, the brain, there is no sensory experience, no pain, and no Problem Patient with Pain. As described in the syllogism above, brain, body, and mind are one; we are our brains. For instance, A-beta, A-delta, and C-nociceptive fibers from the periphery of the body do not transmit, touch, vibratory sensation, heat, cold, pain, or any other specific sensation. Initiation of an action potential by appropriate peripheral stimulation results in the transmission of uninterpreted information. This information is relayed through the thalamus, where incoming data may be influenced or even inhibited by descending cortical activity. The cortical influence on the input is determined by the adaptive state of the individual. If the input is not inhibited, it ultimately activates the parietal and somatosensory-somatomotor cortex. In the parietal cortex, this information is correlated, analyzed, synthesized, integrated, and interpreted, which requires memory, a distributed cortical function.[10, 19, 34, 56] The current adaptive context of the individual, correlated with memory, gives meaning to the information received. This process can only occur in the presence of conscious cortical functioning, and as Edelman has clearly demonstrated, consciousness requires memory. There can be no experience of pain, except reflexive withdrawal, without memory, because there can be no consciousness without memory. The Problem Patient with Pain, in all probability, is presenting metaphorically a memorial event. He or she is consciously aware of the painful affect but not the underlying memory that provokes it. Every reportable experience, painful or otherwise, requires activation of cortical neuronal groups in a conscious individual. When heat or pinprick applied to the periphery results in a nerve action potential, the subsequent sensation is felt not in the periphery but in the conscious cortex as a consequence of activated neuronal groups in the somatotopic, cortical representation of the stimulated peripheral area. This, of course, is clearly consistent with the results of neurosurgical stimulation of the somatosensory cortex in alert patients in attempts to detect epileptic foci. It is also consistent with the complaints of amputees with phantom limb phenomenon.[11]

Hallucinatory experiences, particularly auditory hallucinations, are well known. Hallucinations can occur in any sensory modality, although less frequently and less often recognized than auditory disturbances. Sensations reflecting hallucinatory phenomena may be olfactory, gustatory, visual, and tactile. Hallucinations are not pathognomonic of schizophrenia or any other major mental disorder.[3] Hallucinations are well known to follow head injury and may occur in any or all sensory modalities and submodalities. Hallucinations result from activation of identifiable cortical areas as demonstrated in studies with positron emission tomography scans.[43, 44] Phantom limb phenomena are somatosensory hallucinations probably caused by excessive reorganizational activity in the somatosensory-somatomotor cortex in the receptive field of the amputated limb. Numbness and tingling of an extremity or other body area may occur as an aura to seizures arising in the parietal or other cortical areas. They may also occur as a consequence of adaptively initiated cortical activity. Neuronal group activity may be initiated by adaptive imperatives and associated imagery.[1, 49] This may give rise to sensory phenomena which develop within parietal or other cortical areas. The neural activity is restricted to those areas, although experienced as located in the periphery.[3, 33, 43–45] The individual has no way of differentiating between activation arising within the cortex from activation evoked from the periphery, because all conscious experience is sensed within the cortex.[52] When an individual patient or physician insists that a sensation or pain is coming from "out there"—hand, leg, chest, or other body part—in the absence of corroborative information, the patient and the physician may be unwittingly colluding in an effort to make a somatic delusion a private reality. This adaptively initiated, image-driven cortical activity may also be associated with or may precipitate limbic activity, which then drives the hypothalamic-pituitary-adrenocortical axis.[1, 19, 49, 54] It is the latter situation that creates the peripheral autonomic changes so frequently misconstrued as pathogenic and labeled as reflex sympathetic dystrophy. This is what makes reflex sympathetic dystrophy, as Ochoa says, "a dangerous diagnosis to be given." It is dangerous because, in this situation, the Problem Patient with Pain is presenting an adaptively initiated, image-driven, physiologic response that has been misdiagnosed as pathology.[1, 54] Stellate ganglion blocks, sympathectomies, and other interventions are less than useful for such patients; they are harmful physiologically and psychologically.

Forty-one years ago, Holmes and Wolff conducted a well-documented study in which they evaluated Problem Patients with Pain, specifically low back pain. They were able to demonstrate that the emotional state of their subjects—disturbing affects, wishes, fantasies, and recollections—provoked pain complaints and electric activity in the muscles about which they complained. No neuromusculoskeletal or other pathology was identified as a cause of their complaints.[29]

The following case provides a dramatic illustration of the validity of the thesis offered by Holmes and Wolff more than 40 years ago and Ochoa's more recent warning.

A 42-year-old woman presented with complaints of severe pain in the right hand after a laceration of the tips of her index and middle fingers. Complaints of pain were associated with coolness in the hand and a report of changes in color. She had become a Problem Patient with Pain and had seen numerous physicians. She had injured her hand at work and been unemployed and essentially nonfunctional for more than 3 years. She was diagnosed as having reflex sympathetic dystrophy, which led to a dozen sympathetic blocks without placebo control and without consistent response. Sympathectomy was being considered, and she was referred for evaluation. Collateral information indicated that she was a battered wife. She insisted, however, that everything in her life was fine except for the "pain." An extensive interview was conducted, using a format similar to that described by Holmes and Wolff but with modern electronic equipment and computers. Physiologic parameters were real-time recorded from a computer monitor and videotaped. All physiologic parameters were stabilized through biofeedback relaxation techniques and were bilaterally symmetric at the time the interview was initiated. As the interview proceeded, the patient was asked about her relationship with her husband. She responded with an idealistic description that clinically suggested active defensiveness and unconscious denial of reality. Within a few seconds of the inquiry about her husband, the skin temperature of the dominant, injured right hand dropped precipitously, heart rate and respiration increased, and surface electromyographic recordings over the right trapezius demonstrated significantly increased voltage. At the same time, the patient indicated, through a pressure gauge, the presence of severe pain. This woman clearly illustrated how adaptively initiated imagery, a recall of the relationship with her husband, provoked somatic and autonomic responses that had come to be medically designated as characteristic of organic pathology. Her difficulties would never be ameliorated by the medical interventions contemplated. Again, we need to note that the history that one does not know is often the history that one needs.

Two other cases provide us with similar information but from different perspectives.

A 29-year-old woman was examined by the author and a resident in an outpatient neurology clinic. She had presented with complaints of severe numbness, tingling, and pain in her hands. The only clinical finding was a bilateral-glove hypoesthesia. Electrophysiologic studies were normal. She was a refugee from a war-torn Latin American country and did not speak English. During my interview, her interpreter, a relative, stated that she had left her 9-year-old daughter behind. I directed the interpreter to have the patient look at me and tell me in Spanish, without interpretation, exactly what her daughter looked like the last time she saw her. This young woman immediately became extremely anxious and restless and actively resisted this request. She indicated that it was not related to why she was being seen, a common response of patients in this predicament. Nevertheless, she complied. As she looked me in the eyes and began to speak, her face became contorted, her eyes watered, and she quickly collapsed, sobbing, in a chair. Her symptoms disappeared, and at subsequent follow-up, she was significantly improved emotionally, in response to the initiation of efforts at reuniting her with her daughter. This young woman provides a vivid example of the interactive relation between unresolved personal issues, imagery, and verbal complaints presented as neurologic symptoms.

A 39-year-old woman was referred by her orthopedist because of depression. She also complained of numbness, tingling, and pain in her hands. She had already been the benefactor, or victim, of bilateral carpal tunnel releases. Her symptoms remained unchanged, and she was referred for consultation and treatment. She was depressed and angry about how she felt taken advantage of in her marriage and by everyone with whom she interacted, including her children. A significant element of her past history was that she had been sent at age 10 to live with an aunt when her mother died. The patient reported that she was isolated and treated abusively in the aunt's family. She specifically recalled having her hands tied to a desk, where she was forced to sit 4 hours a night after school and an equivalent time on the weekends. In late adolescence, she ran away. The recollection of her history was painful and provoked increased somatic complaints along with feelings of hopelessness and despair. After several weeks on treatment with fluoxetine, 20 mg a day, she began to feel more assertive and verbally aggressive when she felt disadvantaged. She spoke up at gatherings and pressed for her own position. Her complaints of numbness, tingling, and pain in her hands disappeared. She was essentially symptom-free; however, her newly expressed assertiveness greatly disturbed her. She became fearful and uncertain in her relationships with others and anxious that she would lose control of her aggressiveness. Even though her original presenting symptoms were eliminated, apparently as a result of the medication, she stopped taking the medication. She could not manage the significant changes in her adaptive style. The complaints of numbness, tingling, and hand pain slowly reappeared, and she returned to her quiet, compliant, chronically resentful self. Fluoxetine has an effect, almost exclusively, on the cortex, as this patient demonstrates. Her complaints were somatosensory hallucinations resulting from memorial activation of the somatotopic representation of the hands in the somatosensory cortex. I am convinced, from many experiences such as that demonstrated by this woman, that these symptoms serve an adaptive purpose; they help the patient maintain control over powerful, potentially disruptive affects that threaten them with disorganization and more crippling dysfunction.

It is usually the suppressed, underlying rage of these patients that provokes our adverse reactions to them as patients. Unless we can tolerate their affects and understand what they are communicating, we are at risk of promoting them as Problem Patients with Pain because as we unconsciously respond to the helplessness and futility they create in us, we are likely to resort to unwarranted interventions.

Those Problem Patients with Pain whose complaints repeatedly defy legitimate diagnosis but are easily described with ambiguous diagnoses, are serving notice to us that their complaints probably do not mean what they seem to mean. If these patients are to be understood, one must consider their symptoms as somatic metaphors. A "pain in the neck" may be due to an injury to the neck, but it may also be a reference to the conflicts in a painful marital or other relationship. To say that someone gives us a headache or makes us sick or uptight is a diagnostic statement that we all understand but too frequently ignore. Verbal complaints of this nature are rarely understood by the patient or the physician for what they actually mean. These complaints are important because they are the vehicle for the doctor–patient relationship.[37, 57, 58] Because the patient's focus is on the body, any attempts to shift this frame of reference to the intrapsychic or interpersonal provokes a feeling in the patient that he or she is being dismissed and that his or her complaints are not being taken seriously. This type of response is a rationalization for the defensive nature of their complaints. It is an adaptive effort to coerce the physician to support their somatic delusion. The suggestion to the patient of an alternative clinical hypothesis must be conducted with great tact, skill, and understanding. Under the best of circumstances, suggesting an alternative hypothesis is likely to be met with marked but quiet resistance. These complaints or symptoms are critical to the patient's functioning, and tactless efforts to clarify their real significance often result in overt hostility. Therefore, it may be very tempting to slip into supporting the patient's somatic delusion. If the patient refuses to consider alternative diagnostic possibilities in the face of inadequate support for his or her hypothesis, we must consider the likelihood that this Problem Patient with Pain is presenting a somatic delusion.

We all offer rationalizations for our actions. These rationalizations may consist of complaints that one is injured and therefore unable to function. Rationalization is a left brain function used to justify feelings, motivation, and behavior. Rationalizations are on the same spectrum as delusions. A rationalization that is so important and firmly held that no other explanation can be considered is probably a delusion. Many back, neck, and other somatic pain complaints fall into this category; they are somatic delusions. The studies of Sperry, Gazzaniga, and others in split-brain patients have demonstrated that an individual may be given written instructions through the right brain, but the left brain is unaware of the instructions. When the person is asked what he or she is doing, in response to the right brain instruction, they reply with a rationalization. In other words, he or she confabulates. He or she tries to match the behavior that he or she has observed in himself or herself rationally with an explanation for a motivation that he or she would find acceptable. He or she cannot verbally express the real reason for the behavior because the left brain does not know the motivation. The left brain provides a "verbal because" for the right brain information when the left brain is asked about the behavior. The left brain is, of course, aware of the behavior but just not aware of the instruction that provided the motivation.[22–25, 51] This type of rationalization has been demonstrated repeatedly in split-brain studies and also in hypnosis with posthypnotic suggestion. In the same way that the patient with split brain does not recognize the source of their motivation, a patient with an adaptively initiated, image-driven somatosensory hallucination; pain; numbness; tingling; or weakness does not recognize the source of his or her motivation for these somatic experiences and therefore rationalizes them. When the rationalization, which does not conform to clinical reality, becomes firmly entrenched, the position of the patient and his or her fixed idea about the nature of the trouble is clearly a somatic delusion. When patient and physician share this position, we are confronted with a therapeutic misalliance or *folie à deux*. If we, as physicians, participate with the patient in marketing their delusional constructions, we are ensuring the continuity of complaints in our Problem Patient with Pain. As physicians, our first responsibility is to do no harm. If the Problem Patient with Pain wishes to market his or her somatic delusions, there is usually ready access to the legal profession. Many attorneys make a living marketing somatic delusions.[30]

CONCLUSION

The brain is the organ of adaptation, and we are our brains; the mind is what the brain does, and the body performs as the adapting brain directs. Without the brain, there is no adaptation, and there is, of course, no person and no Problem Patient with Pain. The lowest levels of the sensory system abstract information from both the external and internal environment according to rules that have evolved over time and have served adaptation. How information is received and processed and the meaning given to it are determined by the individual history of the particular brain, that is, the particular individual. This history is available in the individual's memory.[19, 50] Abstraction of sensory information becomes a signal that is transmitted and automatically elicits responses at a synaptic, cellular level as the brain naturally but unconsciously uses this information for adaptive purposes. This signal or information influences behavior but has no meaning and cannot be articulated or verbalized until it is consciously processed by the left hemisphere. The left hemisphere is the side of the brain that offers the "because." As we have seen, this "because" does not have to coincide with the actual factors that give rise to the motivation for a particular behavior or complaint, because those factors are probably not consciously known to the patient.

As mentioned earlier, nociceptive and other receptors, specialized nerve endings that elicit nerve action potentials in response to pressure, heat, cold, and noxious energy and their associated pathways, do not transmit heat, cold, or pain. They transmit information that provokes unconscious brain activity, leading to often subtle, automatic changes in adaptation. If the rate of rise or amount of signal information is sufficient, regardless of its source, internal or external, the experience may become conscious and, in the proper context, painful.[60, 66] Thoughts, images, ideas, or feelings arise from either external or internal signals coupled with memories and are as capable of stimulating a somatotopic sensory or motor cortical neuronal group as are peripheral receptors. That is, somatotopically organized sensations can arise within the brain without a peripheral source, and this finding cannot be overemphasized. When patients present with various complaints that cannot be specifically identified as arising in the periphery through use of the usual or even highly technical procedures, it does not mean that we need to repeat those procedures incessantly or that the patient is lying, that is, he or she is not actually having the experience about which he or she complains. If we fail to consider the coherent integration and function of the mind, body, and brain, we may be led into an abyss of confusion in the clinical evaluation of patients, particularly with regard to neurologic and general medical complaints and specifically with regard to evaluation of the Problem Patient with Pain.

To reach the highest degree of medical probability with respect to verbal complaints of pain in an individual patient with general medical or peripheral nerve type symptoms, a detailed and definitive history of the individual, as well as physiologically specific diagnostic studies, must be obtained. In the case of sensory complaints, the patient must have the opportunity for extensive neurophysiologic assessment that evaluates peripheral performance and the integrity of the peripheral nervous system. Second, the individual patient has to be understood as an adapting person with a given history, considering how he or she functions and views the world, not merely as someone with verbal symptoms or complaints. When the physician knows the individual, he or she can make effective, appropriate medical interventions even in ambiguous situations. Even when we know the patient, further investigation often reveals that the clinical picture is not at all as represented in the patient's verbal complaints of pain. The ambiguity arises from the complexity of the function of the brain and the conflicts the patient is attempting to manage in his or her life. We cannot effectively "manage" the Problem Patient with Pain unless we refuse to collude in the patient's somatic delusion. If we do that, we can possibly come to know what the "pain" really means.

References

1. Achterberg J: Science and the imagination: Physiology and biochemistry. *In* Imagery in Healing: Shamanism and Modern Medicine. (New Science Library). Boston, Shambhala, 1985, pp 113–141
2. Adler G: Helplessness in the helpers. Br J Med Psychol 45:315, 1972
3. Asaad G, Shapiro B: Hallucinations: Theoretical and clinical overview. Am J Psychiatry 143:1088–1097, 1986
4. Beecher HK: Surgery as placebo. JAMA 176:1102–1107, 1961
5. Benson HB, McCallie D: Angina pectoris and the placebo effect. N Engl J Med 300:1424–1429, 1979
6. Bibring GL: Psychiatry and medical practice in a general hospital. N Engl J Med 254:366–372, 1956
7. Boden SD: Abnormal magnetic resonance imaging scans of the cervical spine in asymptomatic individuals. Audiotaped Continuing Education in Orthopedic Surgery, The Orthopedic Audio-Synopsis Foundation, 23:01, April 1991
8. Boden SD, Davis D, Dina T, et al: Abnormal magnetic resonance scans of the lumbar spine in asymptomatic subjects. Journal Bone Joint Surg [Am] 72:403, 1990
9. D'Amour M, Shahani B, Young R, et al: Importance of studying sural nerve conduction and late responses in the evaluation of alcoholic subjects. Neurology 29:1600–1604, 1979
10. DeJong RN: Localization of sensory disorders. *In* The Neurologic Examination. New York, Harper and Row, 1979, pp 78–80
11. DeJong RN: Function and disorders of function of the cerebral cortex. *In* The Neurologic Examination. New York, Harper and Row, 1979, pp 616–617
12. Edelman GM: Summary and historical introduction. *In* Neural Darwinism: The Theory of Neuronal Group Selection. New York, Basic Books, 1987, pp 3–22
13. Edelman GM: Structure function and perception. *In* Neural Darwinism: The Theory of Neuronal Group Selection. New York, Basic Books, 1987, pp 33–37
14. Edelman GM: Cellular dynamics of neural maps. *In* Neural Darwinism: The Theory of Neuronal Group Selection. New York, Basic Books, 1987, pp 105–139
15. Edelman GM: Consciousness and the scientific observer. *In* The Remembered Present: A Biological Theory of Consciousness. New York, Basic Books, 1989, p 22
16. Edelman GM: Neural darwinism. *In* Neural Darwinism: The Theory of Neuronal Group Selection. New York, Basic Books, 1987, pp 43–69
17. Edelman GM: Developmental bases of diversity: The primary repertoire. *In* Neural Darwinism: The Theory of Neuronal Group Selection. New York, Basic Books, 1987, pp 74–104
18. Edelman GM: Synapses as populations: The bases of the secondary repertoire. *In* Neural Darwinism: The Theory of Neuronal Group Selection. New York, Basic Books, 1987, pp 178–204
19. Edelman GM: Categorization and memory. *In* Neural Darwinism: The Theory of Neuronal Group Selection. New York, Basic Books, 1987, pp 240–242
20. Fox AJ, Lin JP, Pinto RS, et al: Myelographic cervical nerve root deformities. Neuroradiology 116:355–361, 1975
21. Frazer JG: The scape goat. *In* The Golden Bough. New York, Macmillan, 1951, pp 31–37
22. Gazzaniga MS: Right hemisphere language following brain bisection: A 20 year perspective. Am Psychol 38:525–537, 1983

23. Gazzaniga MS: The role of language for conscious experience: Observations from split brain man. Prog Brain Res 54:689–696, 1980
24. Gazzaniga MS, LeDoux JE, Wilson DH: Language, praxis and the right hemisphere: Clues to some mechanisms of consciousness. Neurology 27:1144–1147, 1977
25. Gazzaniga MS, Holtzman JD, Smylie CS: Speech without conscious awareness. Neurology 37:682–685, 1987
26. Groves JE: Taking care of the hateful patient. N Engl J Med 298:883–887, 1978
27. Hackett TP: Which patients turn you off? Medical Economics 46:1594–1599, 1969
28. Hitselberger WE, Witten RM: Abnormal myelograms in asymptomatic patients. J Neurosurg 28:204–206, 1968
29. Holmes TH, Wolff HG: Life situations, emotions and backache. Psychosom Med 14:18–33, 1952
30. Huber PW: The science of things that aren't so: Junk science and its origins. In Galileo's Revenge: Junk Science in the Courtroom. New York, Basic Books, 1991, pp 24–38
31. Huber PW: Rights in Collision. Liability: The Legal Revolution and Its Consequences. New York, Basic Books, pp 72–89
32. Johnson AD: The Problem Claim: A Synopsis: An Approach to Earlier Identification, Washington, Department of Labor and Industries, 1977
33. Katims JJ, Naviasky E, Lorenz K, et al: New screening device for assessment of peripheral neuropathy. J Occup Med 28:1219–1221, 1986
34. Kupferman I: Hemispheric asymmetries and the cortical localization of higher cognitive and affective functions. In Kandel ER, Schwartz JH: Principles of Neuroscience, ed 2. New York, Elsevier, 1985, pp 680–681
35. Leonard BE: Ethanol as a neurotoxin. Biochem Pharmacol 36:2055–2059, 1987
36. Lehman LD: Neurologic complications of alcoholism. Postgrad Med 90:165–169, 1991
37. Lipsitt DR: Medical and psychological characteristics of "crocks." Int J Psychiatry Med 1:15–25, 1970
38. Martin F, Peters T: Alcoholic muscle disease. Alcohol Alcohol 20:125–136, 1985
39. Martins AN, Kempe LG, Pikethly DT, et al: Reappraisal of the cervical myelogram. J Neurosurg 27:27–31, 1967
40. Masson EA, Veves A, Fernando D, et al: Current perception thresholds: A new, quick and reproducible method for assessment of peripheral neuropathy in diabetes mellitus. Diabetologia 32:724–728, 1989
41. McRae DL: Asymptomatic intervertebral disc protrusions. Acta Radiol 46:9–27, 1984
42. Mills KR, Ward K, Martin F, et al: Peripheral neuropathy and myopathy in chronic alcoholism. Alcohol Alcohol 21:357–362, 1986
43. Musalek M, Podreka I, Suess E, et al: Neurophysiological aspects of auditory hallucinations: 99m-Tc-hHMPAO-SPECT investigations in patients with auditory hallucinations and normal controls—a preliminary report. Psychopathology 21:275–280, 1988
44. Musalek M, Podreka I, Walter H, et al: Regional brain function in hallucinations: A study of regional cerebral blood flow with 99m-Tc-HMPAO-SPECT in patients with auditory hallucinations, tactile hallucinations and normal controls. Comp Psychiatry 30:99–108, 1989
45. Niewiadomska M, Wochnik-Dyjas D, Czerwosz L: Investigations on the peripheral motor neuron in subjects with alcohol dependence syndrome. Electromyogr Clin Neurophysiol 27:91–97, 1987
46. Ochoa JL: A dangerous diagnosis to be given. European Journal of Pain 12:63–64, 1991
47. Ochoa JL, Verdugo R: Reflex sympathetic dystrophy: Definitions and history of the ideas: A critical review of human studies. In Low PA (ed): The Evaluation and Management of Clinical Autonomic Disorders. Boston, Little, Brown, 1992
48. Ochoa JL: Afferent and sympathetic roles in chronic "neuropathic" pains: Confessions on misconceptions. In Besson JM, Guilbaud G (eds): Lesions of Primary Afferent Fibers as a Tool for the Study of Clinical Pain. Amsterdam, Elsevier, 1991, pp 25–44
49. Restak R: Stress and emotion. In The Brain. New York, Bantam Books, 1984, pp 76–86
50. Restak R: Learning and memory. In The Brain. New York, Bantam Books, 1984, pp 190–191
51. Restak R: The two brains. In The Brain. New York, Bantam Books, 1984, pp 247–265
52. Roland PE, Eriksson L, Stone-Elander S, et al: Mental activity changes the oxidative metabolism of the brain. J Neurosci 8:2373–2389, 1987

53. Rottsberger JT, Buie DH: Counter transference in the treatment of suicidal patients. Arch Gen Psychiatry 30:625–633, 1974
54. Sawchenko PE: Tale of three peptides: Corticotropin-releasing factor-, oxytocin-, and vasopressin-containing pathways mediating integrated hypothalamic responses to stress. *In* McCubbin JA, Kaufman PG, Nemeroff CB (eds): Stress, Neuropeptides and Systemic Disease. New York, Academic Press, 1991, pp 3–17
55. Shapiro AK: A contribution to a history of the placebo effect. Behav Sci 5:109–135, 1960
56. Sherman SM, Koch C: Thalamus. *In* Shepherd GM (ed): The Synaptic Organization of the Brain, ed 3. New York, Oxford University Press, 1990, pp 246–278
57. Shorter E: Doctors and patients at the outset. *In* From Paralysis to Fatigue: A History of Psychosomatic Illness in the Modern Era. New York, The Free Press, 1992, pp 1–24
58. Shorter E: Spinal irritation. *In* From Paralysis to Fatigue: A History of Psychosomatic Illness in the Modern Era. New York, The Free Press, 1992, pp 25–39
59. Skrabanek P: Demarcation of the absurd: Credulity and the craft of medicine. Bostonia Magazine of Culture and Ideas, Boston University, July/August 1991, p 31
60. Stein BE, Price DD, Gazzaniga MS: Pain perception in a man with total corpus callosum transection. Pain 38:51–56, 1989
61. Tauber AI: On pigeons, physicians and placebos. Journal of the Royal Society of Medicine 84:328–331, 1991
62. Voiss DV: The medium and the message. *In* Krueger DW (ed): The Last Taboo: Money, as Symbol and Reality in Psychotherapy and Psychoanalysis. New York, Bruner/Mazell, 1986
63. Weissmann G: The flight into sickness. A review: From Paralysis to Fatigue: A History of Psychosomatic Illness in the Modern Era. (Shorter, Edward). The New Republic 6:38–41, 1992
64. Weseley SA, Sadler B, Katims J: Current perception: Preferred tests for evaluation of peripheral nerve integrity. Transactions, American Society of Artificial Internal Organs 34:188–193, 1988
65. Winnicott DW: Hate in the counter transference. Int J Psychoanal 30:69–74, 1949
66. Yarnitsky D, Simone D, Dotson R, et al: Firing frequency of human C polymodal nociceptors: The effect of rate of rise of noxious heat. Society for Neuroscience Abstracts 15:502.5, 1989

Address reprint requests to

Daniel V. Voiss, MS, MD
ACCESS Consulting Systems Incorporated
2370 N.W. Flanders Street
Portland, OR 97210

THE MYOFASCIAL PAIN SYNDROMES

Norman B. Rosen, MD

There are fewer conditions in clinical practice that have generated more controversy and debate than have those conditions that cause musculoskeletal pain and dysfunction. Because pain is subjective and difficult to measure objectively, alleged *disability* from pain is even harder to assess and, further, is colored by a variety of coexisting or superimposed psychosocial variables and contingencies, including, in particular, secondary gain (financial, emotional, escapism, or otherwise). The possible existence of this latter phenomenon, particularly when litigation or other psychosocial dynamic is involved, has invariably raised an aura of suspicion in the minds of many practitioners around any patient who presents with enigmatic pain of obscure origin and, particularly, with unrelenting chronic pain. As a result, pain treatment protocols have not been standardized and range from simple reassurance ("You have to learn to live with it") to surgery (which often fails to give complete relief) and from validation of the alleged disability to ascribing residual disability to emotional or social factors alone.

Fortunately, during the past decade or so, there has occurred an explosion of information that has allowed us to understand better those myriad conditions that cause musculoskeletal pain and dysfunction and, in particular, the role of myofascial pain and dysfunction in contributing to the clinical problems presented by many of these patients.

The myofascial pain syndromes constitute the largest group of unrecognized and undertreated acute and chronic medical problems in clinical practice and are among the most common overlooked causes of chronic pain and chronic disability in clinical medicine.[30, 82, 96] Although lumped into the larger group of patients with so-called fibrositis by many, clearly this is inappropriate, and the myofascial pain syndromes now stand as independent conditions of enormous importance and with myriad manifestations. (A discussion of the various other conditions that cause musculoskeletal pain, including fibrositis, fibromyalgia, and other

---

From Rehabilitation and Pain Management Associates of Baltimore, Baltimore, Maryland

---

PHYSICAL MEDICINE AND REHABILITATION CLINICS
OF NORTH AMERICA

diseases classified under the general heading of *nonarticular rheumatism* follows in a subsequent section; see "Controversies in Nomenclature.")

No discussion of the role of myofascial pain and dysfunction would be complete without a tribute to the two currently most prolific authors in this field, Janet G. Travell and David G. Simons. Dr. Travell's pioneering and ongoing work in this field[79–81, 86–90] and Dr. Simons' tireless efforts to codify musculoskeletal pain and dysfunction[72–81, 89, 90] and to codify and expand the knowledge base relative to these conditions deserve special tribute, and although there have been other clinical advances in the documentation of the existence of these disorders, mainly the development of the pressure threshold meter by Fischer[20–23] and a better awareness of the role of manual medicine techniques by Cyriax,[14, 15] Mennell, Lewit,[44–46] Maitland,[47] Greenman,[32] and others, these two individuals deserve special merit and attention in helping us to understand better the many aspects of the myofascial pain syndromes.

DIAGNOSTIC CONSIDERATIONS

Because of the paucity of objective laboratory studies available to document the existence of these disorders, the diagnosis must rely entirely on the clinical history and the performance of a careful physical examination, not only looking for static abnormalities of muscle and joint that may be present but also assessing the dynamic forces and imbalances operant under both loaded and unloaded conditions. More important, the role of muscle imbalances between groups of muscles, in both loaded and unloaded conditions, must be assessed.

The physical examination often reveals only subtle clinical findings, including a sensation of muscular ropiness, or hardening, of the involved muscles or the finding, within the muscle, of a localized area of increased resistance to palpation (the so-called taut band) in which there is usually found an area of local tenderness that on compression often duplicates the patient's complaints.[88–90] Snapping or needling the taut band often results in a local fasciculation that has been called the *local twitch response*.[88] This local twitch response has been shown by Dexter and Simons,[16] Hong,[36] and others[26] to be spinal cord mediated and is unique to the myofascial pain syndromes. The area of local tenderness within the taut band has been called the *trigger point area*,[88] because of the unique ability of this area not only to cause local pain and tenderness but to trigger referred pain and tenderness elsewhere. The referral patterns thus generated are uniquely characteristic for each myofascial pain syndrome, and each muscle has its own unique referral pattern, which allows the clinician who is aware of these referral patterns to track down the myofascial source of that referral pattern. It is this aspect of the myofascial pain syndromes (the ability to generate referred pain and tenderness to areas remote from the actual trigger point itself, which is often of greater awareness to the patient than the actual trigger point area itself) that has caused much of the confusion in the diagnosis and management of many musculoskeletal problems.

ROLE OF MYOFASCIAL DYSFUNCTION IN ENIGMATIC PAIN PRESENTATIONS

Table 1 lists the characteristics of myofascial pain and dysfunction. Because many asymptomatic, allegedly normal individuals often present with many apparently identical clinical findings on routine assessment (particularly areas of

Table 1. CHARACTERISTICS OF MYOFASCIAL PAIN

History of local pain and tenderness associated with vague or diffuse complaints of stiffness, aching, gelling, tightness, numbness, tingling, weakness, or coolness in a localized area of the body
Muscular ropiness with localized areas of hardening (taut band)
Areas of localized tenderness within the taut band (the trigger point)
Compression of the trigger point results in referred pain and tenderness to areas remote from that trigger area and can also cause local tenderness
Local twitch response elicited on snapping or needling the taut band
Characteristic pattern of referred pain and tenderness for each trigger point
Weakness of involved muscle or muscles (may be subtle) harboring trigger points
Loss of joint range of motion (may be subtle)
Immediate reversal of weakness and increased range of motion after inactivation of the trigger point
Autonomic components, including vasoconstriction in the area of referral
Epiphenomena: Nerve, tendon, or blood vessel entrapment; deconditioning; psychosocial dysfunction, including anxiety, depression, fear of activity (actophobia or kinesophobia)

tenderness, skeletal asymmetry, subtle muscle weakness and imbalances, nodular-feeling muscles, and subtle or gross restricted range of motion of joints), the significance of these findings in the patient who presents with enigmatic pain or disability has often been challenged and the alleged disability dismissed as being due to psychological factors, secondary gain, or, at best, simple muscular overuse with symptom magnification. Alternatively, because of the unique ability of these syndromes to trigger referred pain and tenderness to areas remote from the source of that referred pain and tenderness and to mimic dysfunction at those sites, there has often occurred a preoccupation on the part of patients, and their practitioners, directed toward the area of referred pain as being the primary source of the dysfunction (as opposed to the myofascial source of that referred pain). It is this failure to recognize that local pain and tenderness may, in fact, be referred from another source located elsewhere (usually myofascial) that has often resulted in misdiagnosis and in the misdirection of therapeutic energies, with predictable "failure of conservative management" and even "failed surgery" often occurring in the wake of such misdirected energies. Indeed, one of the most common causes of so-called failed surgery is the failure to recognize and treat properly the underlying, or coexisting, myofascial pain and dysfunction first.[57, 62, 64, 65] It should be kept in mind that, although myofascial pain and dysfunction may be the primary cause of the presentation, often a myofascial focus may coexist with other conditions and potentiate their dysfunction.* By treating the associated myofascial pain and dysfunction first or at least concurrently, often the practitioner finds that the associated coexisting pathologic problem also responds better to conservative management.[58, 64–66]

The use of local anesthetic blocks, with 1% lidocaine or 0.5% procaine, to differentiate between local pain and tenderness and referred pain and tenderness is a valuable diagnostic procedure, and often a single diagnostic block results in sustained therapeutic improvement (Table 1). Particularly with the patient who alleges disability and who has poor coping skills, it is imperative to recognize and treat underlying myofascial pain and dysfunction prior to ascribing residual

---

* References 55, 59, 62, 63, 72, 73, 89, and 90.

Table 2. PERPETUATING FACTORS

Mechanical, structural, postural	Allergy
Nutritional	Environmental: Equipment, temperature
Metabolic, endocrine	Sleep deprivation
Electrolyte	Anemia
Infection	Emotional stress
Neurocirculatory factors	Other concurrent disease
External compression	(including fibromyalgia)

disability to psychosocial factors alone.[57] With the patient who has poor coping skills, it becomes even more imperative to correct whatever physical disability that is present and to restore the patient to as functional a lifestyle as possible as quickly as possible.[64, 66] It is important for the physician to recognize that disability is multifactorial, and it is often necessary to apportion disability into its component parts to direct treatment properly and restore the individual to as normal a lifestyle as possible.[50, 89, 90]

PERPETUATING FACTORS

The importance of recognizing and treating the associated perpetuating factors that contribute to pain and dysfunction has been stressed by many authors,* and the reader is reminded that treatment of any patient with pain or disability must, by necessity, be comprehensive in nature, paying attention to all of the perpetuating factors, physical and emotional (Table 2). Successful treatment of myofascial pain and dysfunction, therefore, requires not only treatment of the underlying structural and mechanical dysfunctions seen but also addressing of the physical and emotional stressors that aggravate the dysfunction and that perpetuate the disability (see section on treatment).[58]

CONTROVERSIES IN NOMENCLATURE

Another principal cause for the controversy relative to the acceptance of the concepts of myofascial pain and dysfunction has been that the terminology used to define patients having these conditions has been confusing in the literature. The term *fibrositis* in particular has been abused and misunderstood, and the author would agree with Dr. David Simons'[78] recommendation that it no longer be used except in a historical sense.

First defined by Gowers[31] in 1904, fibrositis was applied to a localized form of dysfunction involving the low back (lumbago), which probably was myofascial and mechanical in nature; however, over the course of the years that followed, the term was applied to almost any unexplained musculoskeletal pain problem, including both localized and more generalized forms. The literature in the early 1900s was controversial, relative both to the existence of these clinical conditions as well as to the existence of associated pathologic findings on biopsy studies of apparently both tender areas and trigger point areas.[11, 77, 89] Hench concluded, in

---

* References 55, 72–75, 86, 88–90.

1936, that the nodules of fibrositis "were accessible only to the fingers of faith" and that "fibrositis is a disease that physicians found but surgeons only rarely find."[11, 34] Although, initially, some reports suggested an "inflammatory response" to be present, other studies failed to document any evidence of inflammation, and it would appear that the suffix *itis* is a misnomer, at least on the basis of most pathologic findings. Recent studies have suggested that findings compatible with local hypoxia may be present,[77, 89] but again, it is not clear whether these biopsies were performed in patients who we now recognize as having a more generalized disease (fibromyalgia) or a localized myofascial pain syndrome.

The problem is further compounded by the fact that these enigmatic musculoskeletal pain conditions were considered by many to be psychogenic in nature, and as late as the 1960s and 1970s, most of the major textbooks on the subject of muscle pain syndromes considered fibrositis to be a disease with strong psychogenic overtones.[6, 71, 92, 99, 100] Similarly, the term *psychogenic rheumatism*, which has been applied to many of these patients, depended on the failure of the clinician to make objective findings. These clinicians often dismissed the subtle clinical findings listed in Table 1 as insignificant, and several authors considered the muscular nodules to be merely "herniated fat pads."[6, 11, 71] Although there may in fact be cases of psychogenic rheumatism, this diagnosis should be made only after a thorough search for all other causes of enigmatic pain, including, in particular, myofascial pain and dysfunction, and only after a true psychological basis for the disability is found.

The terms *nonarticular rheumatism, soft tissue disability, tension myalgia*,[85] and *muscle contraction states* also have been applied to this group of cases that present with enigmatic pain involving the musculoskeletal system. Although these terms have some merit from a classification standpoint, they are confusing, misleading, and often too general and imprecise to be of value clinically. In particular, *nonarticular rheumatism* and *soft tissue disability* are imprecise and misleading because the conditions they allude to are often associated with subtle secondary joint dysfunctions, which must be addressed clinically. Similarly, *tension myalgia* and *muscle contraction states* also are imprecise, misleading, and more suggestive (from a terminology standpoint) of psychic dysfunction as the primary cause of the physiologic increase in tone noted clinically, as opposed to physical factors[2] being responsible. The choice of the word *tension* in particular is an unfortunate one, particularly if used in the more global sense initially intended by its authors, because it makes little distinction between physical or emotional factors as being primary and little distinction as to whether the increase in tension is reactive in nature, secondary to some underlying structural or mechanical dysfunction, or a reflection of underlying primary or secondary psychological tension. Obviously, the treatment implications are different in each of these situations, particularly relative to the choice of medication and to the selection of physical or psychosocial treatment approach. In addition, *tension* has definite psychological implications for most people using this term, and because there is in fact a group of patients who indeed have a true psychophysiologic reaction involving the musculoskeletal system due to intense psychological distress, *tension myalgia* is probably better restricted to those cases in which there is a true increase in muscle tone as a result of increased psychological tension. For those individuals in whom the increase in muscle tone is reactive or secondary to underlying physical factors, we have alternative terminology that can better explain the dysfunctions noted, and it would appear more appropriate to confine the use of *tension* to those cases in which psychic tension is playing the predominant role.

Table 3 depicts the multiplicity of names that have been applied to this spectrum of conditions in patients who present with musculoskeletal pain and

Table 3. THE CONFUSING NOMENCLATURE OF MUSCLE PAIN SYNDROMES

Muscular rheumatism	Myofascial trigger area
Nonarticular rheumatism	Myofascial trigger point
Inflammatory rheumatism	Myofascial pain syndromes
Nodular rheumatism	Trigger point disease
Musculorheumatism	Trigger point syndromes
Rheumatic muscle callus	Fibrositis syndromes
Lumbago	Interstitial myofibrositis
Fibrositis	Fibromyalgia
Myofibrositis	Repetitive motion syndrome
Myogelose—gelling	Repetitive strain injury
Muscular hardening	Overuse syndromes
Rheumatic muscle hardening	Overload syndromes
Myalgia	Osteochondrosis
Myogelosis	Chronic fatigue syndrome
Ideopathic myalgia	Work-related chronic myalgia
Myositis	Occupational muscle pain
Fibromyositis	Somatic dysfunction
Polymyalgia rheumatica	Soft tissue disability
Somatic trigger area	Myofascial dysfunction
Rheumatic myalgia	Costochondral syndrome
Psychogenic rheumatism	Levator syndrome
Tension myalgia	Rheumatic pain modulation disorder
Muscle contraction pain	Myofascial pain modulation disorder
Myofascial pain	Chronic myofascial pain disorder

dysfunction. Unfortunately, there is currently no universally accepted terminology, and clearly, to progress in our understanding of musculoskeletal pain and dysfunction, there is a need to adopt a uniform terminology. It is hoped that the classification suggested in Table 4 will allow clinicians to codify more accurately the dysfunctions seen in patients who present with musculoskeletal pain and dysfunction.[62, 77]

Interestingly, the current terms in vogue in the sports medicine literature, as well as in the occupational and Performing Arts medicine literature, include *overuse syndromes*,[28] *repetitive trauma syndromes*, and *repetitive injury or strain syndromes*. Although these terms reflect some of the components of the pathophysiology, they overlook some of the more critical issues that we discuss later in the pathogenesis of many of these overlapping disorders. Unfortunately (and surprisingly), in most of the literature of these specialties, there is still a paucity of information relative to the existence of, and the significance of, the myofascial pain syndromes, and in fact many of these overuse and repetitive trauma syndromes are myofascial pain syndromes but apparently have not been appreciated as such. Further, there is a continued preoccupation in the literature of these subspecialties with apparent local phenomena (of joint, tendon, ligament, nerve, and bursa), without taking into consideration the fact that some of the apparent local dysfunction may in fact be referred from (or colored by) myofascial foci located elsewhere.

Fortunately, over the course of the past 15 years or so, there has been a renewed interest in the group of patients who present with musculoskeletal pain and dysfunction, and this, combined with a proliferation of papers in the literature and newer textbooks on this subject, has refined our understanding of these disorders. Table 4 outlines our current understanding of the classification of these disorders.

THE MUSCLE PAIN DISORDERS

It is probably better to view the entire spectrum of diseases that present with muscular pain as being simply the "muscle pain disorders" (see Table 4).[62, 77] Primary joint dysfunction can often precipitate secondary muscular pain and dysfunction in the muscles that control or move these joints, which may then subsequently develop secondary trigger point phenomena. Alternatively, myofascial dysfunction and imbalances originating within the muscles may create abnormal stresses on the joints that predisposes them, in turn, to dysfunction. Thus, it would appear reasonable to consider articular dysfunction with secondary muscle pain as one clinical entity and myofascial pain with or without secondary joint dysfunction to be a separate entity.

The disease *fibromyalgia*, defined by Yunus in 1981,[101, 102] probably should be considered a separate disease and a primary disease of muscle that is, as yet, of unknown origin. Ongoing research is active in this area to define further the nature of the dysfunction in this condition, which is manifested by widespread pain and tenderness in multiple areas of the body[97, 98] and associated clinical complaints of fatigue and weakness. There is currently experimental evidence that fibromyalgia may be a disease of abnormal energy mobilization,[8, 9, 35] but whether it is due to a viral, allergic, autoimmune, or another process is not clear.[90] The literature suggests that fibromyalgia may be inherited,[52] but its

Table 4. CLASSIFICATION OF MUSCLE PAIN DISORDERS

Primary articular dysfunction with secondary muscular dysfunction
    Inflammatory
    Mechanical, structural
    Autoimmune, connective tissue, vasculitis
    Infectious
    Metabolic, endocrine
Myofascial pain syndrome with or without secondary joint dysfunction
    Independent focus
    Associated with other active process
    Sympathetic-mediated
Fibromyalgia: primary disease of muscle of unknown origin
    ?Inherited defect
    ?Viral
    ?Autoimmune
    ?Allergic
Rheumatic pain modulation disorder
Metabolic, endocrine, electrolyte, or inherited defect
Infectious: viral, bacterial, parasitic, other
Vasculitis, autoimmune, polymyalgia rheumatica, rheumatic-related
Neurologic
    Central disinhibition syndrome: sensory or motor
    Myotonia, paramyotonia
    Viral: poliomyelitis, Guillain-Barré syndrome
    Reflex sympathetic dystrophy
Trauma, postexercise soreness
Neoplasm
Toxic
Psychogenic, tension myalgia, conversion reaction, psychophysiologic reaction of
    the musculoskeletal system
Reactive: tendinitis, bursitis, spasm

predominance in women, its delayed clinical manifestation until puberty or later, and its development (or appearance) after physical or emotional trauma are not explained. Caro,[13] Enestrom,[17] and others have documented a gamma globulin in the skin of many of these patients, suggesting a widespread process of which muscle may merely be one component. There continues to be great controversy over whether fibromyalgia is a disease of peripheral or one of central origin.

The American College of Rheumatology, as a result of a multicenter study, established the current criteria for the diagnosis of fibromyalgia in 1989[97]; they are listed in Table 5.

The reader is cautioned, however, that there are several other conditions that fulfill the current diagnostic criteria to document the existence of fibromyalgia, and merely because someone fulfills the current diagnostic criteria for fibromyalgia does not mean that that individual has fibromyalgia.[62] Table 6 lists some other conditions that should be kept in mind when one is faced with a patient who presents with generalized pain and tenderness in multiple areas of the body. Many of the other conditions listed in Table 4 should also be kept in mind when one is confronted with a patient who presents with widespread symptoms and signs.

The rheumatic pain modulation sleep disorder[51] deserves a special category in the classification, because sleep deprivation alone has been documented by Moldofsky to cause generalized, widespread muscular pain and tenderness and can worsen the pain and fatigue associated with any of the other categories.

The clinician should also always keep in mind other causes of muscular pain, including muscle pain associated with and secondary to vasculitis, polymyositis, or other rheumatic disease; the nonspecific myalgias associated with a variety of viral, parasitic, or other infections; toxic exposure; or neuroendocrine dysfunction. Other causes of muscle pain are listed in Table 4.

Although fatigue is the primary complaint of individuals who present with the chronic fatigue syndrome, many of these individuals have widespread complaints and tenderness sufficient to satisfy the criteria of fibromyalgia but do not have fibromyalgia. Similarly, the reader is also reminded that multifocal myofascial pain syndromes, which may just happen to coexist,[61] may also satisfy the criteria for the existence of fibromyalgia but again are not necessarily this condition.

Table 5. CURRENT DIAGNOSTIC CRITERIA OF THE AMERICAN COLLEGE OF RHEUMATOLOGY FOR THE CLASSIFICATION OF FIBROMYALGIA

History of widespread pain, present for at least 3 months
The presence of tenderness in 11 of 18 tender point sites on digital palpation
    (approximate force of 4 kg)
  Occiput: bilateral, at the suboccipital muscle insertions
  Lower cervical: bilateral, at the anterior aspects of the intertransverse spaces at
    C5–7
  Trapezius: bilateral, at the midpoint of the upper border
  Supraspinatus: bilateral, at origins, above the scapular spine near the medial
    border
  Second rib: bilateral, at the second costochondral junction, just lateral to the
    junctions on the upper surface
  Lateral epicondyle: bilateral, 2 cm distal to the epicondyles
  Gluteal: bilateral, in upper outer quadrants of the buttocks and anterior fold of
    muscle
  Greater trochanter: bilateral, posterior to the trochanteric prominence
  Knee: bilateral, at the medial fat pad proximal to the joint line

Table 6. CONDITIONS THAT FULFILL THE CRITERIA OF THE AMERICAN COLLEGE OF RHEUMATOLOGY FOR THE CLASSIFICATION OF FIBROMYALGIA

Fibromyalgia
Rheumatic pain modulation disorder
Multifocal myofascial pain syndromes
Chronic fatigue syndrome
Psychogenic rheumatism, hysteria, malingering, symptom magnification disorders, somatization syndromes

Furthermore, it has been pointed out by Simons and others, that many of the tender points of fibromyalgia may in fact be due to, or in the referral area of, myofascial trigger points.[76, 78] Before tenderness is ascribed to a tender point of fibromyalgia, potential myofascial foci in adjacent muscles should be sought and eradicated to ensure that the tender areas are in fact not referred tenderness from undiscovered trigger points.

CLASSIFICATION OF MYOFASCIAL PAIN SYNDROMES

The myofascial pain syndromes have traditionally been viewed as being single muscle syndromes,[72–81, 86–90] although, clearly, dysfunction in one muscle is often accompanied by dysfunction in the other muscles of the myotatic unit, including the co-movers, the synergists, the antagonists, and the proximal stabilizers.[89, 90] The importance of assessing the other muscles of the myotatic or functional unit for evidence of myofascial dysfunction cannot be overstressed, particularly when one is faced with a patient who has persistent dysfunction in one region, presumably on the basis of a single muscle disorder. The apparent single muscle dysfunction may, in fact, be due to dysfunction in other muscles of the functional unit, unknown to the patient and found only after a careful search by the clinician. Muscles work in pairs or in groups, and the single muscle dysfunction seen may in fact be *reactive* and secondary to dysfunction in another muscle or unit of the myofascial network located elsewhere. There are key muscles in every part of the body that predispose that region to dysfunction, and these muscles have been called the *gateway muscles*[62] because, once discovered and treated, they invariably open the gate to successful treatment of the more apparent single muscle dysfunctions (see section "The Gateway Muscles"). A complete assessment for static and dynamic postural abnormalities and for the mechanical forces that affect these abnormalities should always be performed to understand better just why a single muscle syndrome occurs, particularly when one is faced with a resistant or refractory pain problem.

Although for didactic purposes it is important to recognize the characteristics of the various single muscle syndromes together with their unique patterns of referred pain and tenderness, more often than not multiple muscles are in fact involved and prone to the development of their own unique myofascial pain syndromes. Whether this involvement of multiple muscle groups is due to the well-known phenomenon of spread of myofascial pain and dysfunction or whether this is merely a function of simultaneous breakdown of borderline functioning tissues is not known, and research is necessary to understand the so-called trigger of dysfunction that causes the process in the first place. Further, the clinical presentation is in fact usually a complex one, with multiple patterns of referred pain present and multiple sources of musculoskeletal dysfunction noted.

Table 7. CLASSIFICATION OF MYOFASCIAL PAIN SYNDROMES

Single Muscle Involvement
Focal Involvement (two or more muscles are involved around a single joint)
Regional Involvement (two or more muscles and two or more joints are involved in a
  single region of the body)
Multifocal or Multiregional Involvement (two or more apparently unrelated regions of
  the body are involved)
Generalized Involvement
  Primary muscle (fibromyalgia, other inherited genetic defect)
  Secondary muscle (thyroid deficiency; vitamin deficiency; other hormonal,
    nutritional, or endocrine dysfunction; mechanical; structural; postural;
    vasculitis; sleep deprivation; polyarticular dysfunction)

The propensity for myofascial foci to spread and to develop satellite trigger points in adjacent muscles, synergistic muscles, or other muscles of the myofascial network[62] or chain,[33] which can then in turn serve to set off independent autonomous foci of myofascial dysfunction elsewhere, is one of the more puzzling and as yet undefined areas of research. Just as there are referred sensory phenomena and autonomic phenomena, there may also well be referred motor phenomena that occur in a reflex fashion that may in fact sensitize other muscles to develop myofascial foci and breakdown. This may in fact be a possible mechanism responsible for the clinical observation of spread of myofascial pain and dysfunction.

Thus, it is clinically important to view the myofascial syndromes from the standpoint of five separate categories (Table 7).[61] Particularly with the patient who has generalized pain, it is important to break the problem down into component parts, as suggested by Table 7, and to try to solve one problem at a time, one area at a time.[61]

The stages of myofascial pain (Table 8) have been commented on by other authors[89, 90] and are not reviewed here, except to point out that there are many asymptomatic individuals who do in fact have muscular nodularity, subtle weakness, and subtle loss of range of motion but no local tenderness or referred pain elicited on compression of the associated potential trigger point area. These patients may in fact have a prelatent phase of dysfunction in the eventual development of myofascial pain and dysfunction.[62] Further research is required to comment further, however.

Table 8. STAGES OF MYOFASCIAL PAIN

Normal: Pain-free, no nodules or ropiness
Prelatent: Pain-free; ropiness or tightness (or both) may be present; no referred
  symptoms; LTR may or may not be present, but no pain can be elicited
Latent: Asymptomatic except for local ropiness and tenderness; LTR may be
  present; referred pain on manipulation of the latent trigger point; local tightness
  of muscle groups and subtle restricted motion or weakness may be present
Active, activity-related: Ropiness and local tenderness present; a taut band with an
  associated LTR present; characteristic pattern of referral; symptoms occur only
  with activity
Active, constant: Symptoms occur both at rest and with activity; other findings as
  per Table 1

LTR = local twitch response.

THE GATEWAY MUSCLES

When one attempts to assess the patient who presents with myofascial pain and dysfunction, it is important not to be misled by the fact that an individual has an apparent single muscle syndrome. Each region of the body has its own unique gateway muscle[62] that may predispose that part of the body to the development of a variety of single muscle syndromes. Unsuccessful treatment of the single muscle syndrome should invariably prompt a search for other areas of myofascial pain in other muscles of the myotatic unit and should also prompt a search for a focus of myofascial pain in the gateway muscle group. The gateway muscle may harbor a latent or active trigger point or may merely be tight because of other reasons, including old apparently resolved but incompletely healed trauma, or shortening due to postural or other factors. For the most part, these muscles tend to be the flexors and the internal rotators.[59]

Thus, with apparent single-muscle neck, trapezius, or levator scapulae dysfunction, one should always conduct a search for myofascial foci in not only the other extensors of the neck but also the flexors of the neck and shoulders, including the internal rotators. Thus, a search for myofascial dysfunction in the sternocleidomastoid, the scalenii, the subscapularis, and the pectoralis muscle groups should always be performed when faced with a patient who has persistent neck, dorsal spine, or posterior shoulder dysfunction, particularly with a forward head, anterior-rounded shoulder position.[89, 90] Similarly, in the low back, apparent single muscle dysfunction of the gluteii, paraspinous muscles, or other muscles simulating sacroiliac dysfunction should always prompt a search for coexisting dysfunction in the abdominal muscles; the hip flexors, including the iliopsoas and rectus femoris; and the quadratus lumborum,[89, 90] which is a lateral flexor and stabilizer of the spine. Persistent foot, ankle, and leg dysfunction should always prompt a search for dysfunction in the tibialis posterior or flexor digitorum longus, and persistent knee and anterior thigh dysfunction should lead to a search for dysfunction in the hamstrings and the adductors, particularly the adductor magnus.[89, 90]

OVERUSE VERSUS OVERLOAD

It is the paradox of the myofascial pain syndromes that these syndromes occur in muscles that have been both overused as well as in those muscles that have been underused. In addition, these syndromes develop in a setting of misuse, abuse, and disuse. Clearly, the common factor in the development of these syndromes in these various situations is not one of use but rather one of exceeding of a "critical load."[62] The term *overuse* is much too restrictive and misleading in attempts to understand the pathophysiology of the development of most of these clinical syndromes, because it does not take into consideration the muscle dysfunction that can also occur as a result of improper use, disuse, or frank abuse. Furthermore, the term does not take into consideration other critical factors, such as the varying load imposed on muscles as a result of faulty positioning, malalignment of forces, underlying joint dysfunction, or a variety of external environmental considerations. In all these situations, something occurs in the muscle in response to a relatively or absolutely abnormal load that is imposed on the muscle at any particular time, which results in the muscle's fatiguing prematurely and failing once this critical load has been exceeded.[62] Myofascial foci and trigger points develop at a point at which muscles are no longer capable of handling the load and doing the job required of them, perhaps as a result of a physiologic protective mechanism gone awry, with both peripheral and central manifestations occurring.

Although overuse is certainly one component leading to the development of myofascial pain and dysfunction, conceptually it is more important to consider a variety of forces at work, because there are therapeutic implications in terms of our ability to modify or modulate these forces.[59] Rather than merely prescribing rest for presumed overuse, it is incumbent on the practitioner to correct the other factors that may be contributing to the premature fatigue and breakdown of muscles. Although rest is certainly one of the primary therapeutic recommendations for any acute pain state, this recommendation for rest need not be absolute because with complete rest come disuse, further shortening and weakening of muscles, and the propensity for the development of additional myofascial dysfunction due to these factors.

Other avenues for treatment become more apparent when one conceptualizes that the pathophysiology is one of overload of muscles rather than simple overuse. Overload of muscles can occur as a result of a variety of factors, including not only overuse but also malalignment of tissues; poor technique; improper use; inadequate stretching before, during, and after use (lack of warm-up or cool-down); equipment failure; and temperature abnormality. Overload may also result from other environmental factors, including inappropriate work stations or other faultily ergonomically designed equipment causing improper postures, and worn-out or poor equipment and playing surfaces. Other physical and emotional stressors can also contribute to premature fatigue, breakdown, and dysfunction. Each of these factors, if present, should be adequately addressed and corrected simultaneously with the recommendation for rest. This allows the patient a more rapid return to function or work despite residual pain and dysfunction, with his or her tissues at risk better protected to handle the loads required of them (through the use of elastic supports; better training; more flexibility; stronger, proper medication; better ergonomically designed work stations and equipment; warmer environment; proper technique; and less intense work sessions in fixed or faulty postures).

The myofascial pain syndromes are thus better conceptualized as overload syndromes,[59, 62, 63] and overuse is merely one component of a complex process that contributes to the eventual breakdown and dysfunction seen clinically (Table 9).

METABOLIC STUDIES

The issue of just what is occurring at the muscle level is not entirely resolved, although clearly, recent studies have suggested that there are findings consistent with local hypoxia in the area of involvement.[77, 89] Simons, Travell, and others have suggested that the trigger point area occurs in an area of "metabolic distress,"[77, 89] which probably develops as the result of the body's inability to handle the critical load mentioned in the last section. As a result, muscle dysfunction occurs and persists because of a combination of factors, including an increased local energy demand and a decreased energy supply to that area. This increased energy demand occurs at a point at which the muscle work reaches a critical level (the critical load), at which time the supply of oxygen is diminished locally through a variety of local interactions designed to be protective and presumably under sympathetic nervous system control. Simons[77] has suggested that this combination of factors could produce a self-sustaining cycle, initiated by

Table 9. FACTORS AFFECTING THE CRITICAL LOAD

Alignment, structure, posture
Static and dynamic loading forces
"Use" syndromes
Hyperlaxity
Balance between agonist and antagonist
Internal milieux and muscle "set" factors
Length-tension relation
Nutrition
Energy supply
Circulation
Sympathetic nervous system
Temperature
Other perpetuating factors (see Table 2)
Psychosocial modulators
External milieux and factors
Physical and emotional stresses
Environmental factors
Temperature
Coexisting entrapment neuropathy

a leak or release of calcium from an injured or otherwise damaged sarcoplasmi reticulum. This would result in a localized contraction of the muscle fibers (possibly designed to be protective) and could result in the formation of the taut band perceived clinically. This localized contraction, however, is associated with a further increase in local metabolic demands, and this increase in metabolic demand, in turn, compromises the adenosine triphosphate energy supply of the sarcoplasmic reticulum and results in a perpetuating cycle of pain and muscle contraction. Physiologically, there may also occur, at the spinal cord level, a variety of reactive responses involving the wide dynamic neurons, perhaps in an effort to modulate the dysfunction, which may in turn activate peripheral responses, perhaps mediated through the sympathetic nervous system. The result is the development of a taut band, manifested by increased local tissue compliance, local hypoxia, and abnormal local metabolic dysfunction, with triggering of central influences that serve to further sensitize and perpetuate the peripheral tissues, thus setting the stage for spread of dysfunction.

Muscles, of course, require an energy system to function adequately, and anything that interferes with the energy supply to the muscle can result in potential dysfunction, including impairment of the circulation due to intrinsic factors (sympathetic nervous system, vasoactive peptides) or extrinsic ones (elastic garters, compression bandages, brassiere straps, or constricting garments). Cold's well-known adverse effect on muscle function should also be kept in mind, and the beneficial effect of external supports may be a function of several factors at work, including increased warmth in the area of the involved muscle.

REFERRED PAIN

Although it was Kellgren,[37] in 1938, who first documented the existence of referred pain and referred tenderness emanating from specific focal areas of muscles, it was through the efforts of subsequent investigators, including Travell, Kelly, Gutstein-Good, Sola, and others, who codified the existence of these multiple patterns of referred pain and tenderness in essentially every muscle of the body. The exact mechanism concerning the pathways responsible for referred pain and the mechanisms causing it are still not known, and the reader is referred to other reviews discussing possible mechanisms responsible for the development of this phenomenon.[76, 77, 89]

In his initial article citing seven case studies, Kellgren[37] pointed out that muscles contained areas of localized tenderness that caused referred pain to other tissues more remote from the source of that referred pain. Furthermore, he pointed out that there were both referred pain and referred tenderness in the area of referral. After a local anesthetic block to the area of referral, the localized tenderness, but not the pain, was abolished. On anesthetizing the more proximal site of localized tenderness, however, not only the tenderness at the site of the injection but also both the referred tenderness and pain in the area of referral were abolished. Furthermore, he pointed out that the pathways conducting pain and tenderness were obviously different from the better-known dermatomal and neurotomal pathways and that the referred tenderness was generally perceived to be deeper and more diffuse than the more superficial pathways associated with dermatomal or neurologic dysfunction. The referred pain was also perceived to be of a different quality and was reported to be burning or aching, in contrast to the sharper pain of more superficial pathways.

In May 1952, Travell and Rinzler, in coining the phrase *myofascial pain syndrome*,[88] pointed out the findings that were to be the cornerstones in the diagnosis of myofascial pain and dysfunction: (1) There were trigger areas located in myofascial structures capable of causing and maintaining pain cycles indefinitely; (2) the trigger point could generate impulses that bombarded the central nervous system and gave rise to referred pain in areas remote from that trigger point; (3) pain was set off whenever a trigger area was stimulated by pressure, needling, heat, cold, or any motion that stretched the structure containing the trigger area; (4) there was a resistance to stretch, leading to a subtle shortening of the affected muscle, with associated limitation of motion and weakness; (5) these trigger points were often associated with vasoconstriction or other autonomic effects that were *limited* to the reference zone of pain; (6) the trigger point, at one particular spot, gives rise to a remarkably constant pattern of referred pain from person to person; and (7) this constancy of pattern enables one to use a known reference pattern of referred pain to locate the myofascial source of that referred pain. Furthermore, they pointed out that because techniques directed at abolishing the trigger point, such as local anesthetic block, terminated the painful episode both at the trigger area and at the area of referred pain, clearly the factor causing the trigger point in the first place was not the factor responsible for keeping it going. The ability of the trigger area with its associated pain pattern to persist long after the precipitating cause of that trigger point had vanished and to function autonomously and independently of the source of that trigger point was the unique factor responsible for perpetuating the pain and dysfunction.

The ability of trigger points to set up satellite trigger points in adjacent or remote muscles or in other muscles of the myotatic unit is currently being investigated, as is the mechanism of referred pain. It is the ability of myofascial pain and dysfunction seemingly to spread either through as-yet-undefined referral mechanisms or as a result of direct interference with function of other tissues (nerve, blood vessel, or other musculotendinous entrapment) that has generated much of the confusion in the understanding of the role of myofascial pain and dysfunction in the first place. Research is active in these areas of referred sensory and motor phenomena. From a clinical perspective, however, it is important to keep in mind that there may be referred motor as well as sensory phenomena that serve to sensitize the muscles in adjacent and remote areas to develop myofascial pain and dysfunction, and this phenomenon may be responsible for the apparent spread of myofascial pain and dysfunction seen clinically.

PAIN VERSUS DYSFUNCTION

It is beyond the scope of this article to review in depth all of the single muscle syndromes, and the reader is referred to the classic textbooks on myofascial pain and dysfunction by Travell and Simons[89, 90] as well as to other reviews on this subject.[77, 79–81, 87, 88]

It should be pointed out, however, that when the myofascial pain syndromes are discussed, the clinician should keep in mind that he or she is dealing with two distinct clinical phenomena: pain on the one hand and dysfunction of the musculoskeletal unit on the other. These two problems may exist independently or may coexist.[61, 62] Pain may be a reflection of musculoskeletal dysfunction, but musculoskeletal dysfunction can exist in a subclinical pain-free state without interfering with activities of daily living. It is only when the individual attempts to stress his tissues beyond those normal requirements of daily living that breakdown occurs and dysfunction intervenes.

Musculoskeletal dysfunction occurs in those settings where patients have residual tightness and loss of full motion, flexibility, and endurance. Musculoskeletal dysfunction occurs when muscles are tight, weak, out of balance, inefficient, and therefore subject to premature breakdown, premature fatigue, and the development of myofascial pain and overload phenomena. Perhaps the most common cause for recurring acute pain is incomplete rehabilitation, and the most common manifestation of incomplete rehabilitation is residual musculoskeletal tightness and dysfunction that has persisted after an underlying pain problem has been resolved.[61, 78]

The osteopathic literature calls this process of musculoskeletal dysfunction *somatic dysfunction*, and this term includes not only the musculoskeletal dysfunction seen but also the secondary neurologic and neurocirculatory responses called into play, which serve to "reset" or protect the function of these tissues that are dysfunctional or at risk for becoming dysfunctional. Musculoskeletal dysfunction may exist independently in a pain-free state or may occur concurrently with pain. Many of the somatic dysfunctions may in fact harbor unrecognized latent trigger points and may be one of the major precipitating factors that sets the stage for the development of clinical pain and further dysfunction. It is incumbent on the clinician to treat pain and musculoskeletal dysfunction as two separate clinical conditions, particularly in the setting of recurring disability and recurring episodes of pain.

Finally, it should also be pointed out that pain and disability from pain are also two separate issues.[60] Pain from whatever cause should always be interpreted in light of the psychosocial dysfunction also seen. Unfortunately, physicians are often exhorted to deal with impairment and not disability, yet to treat individuals who present with pain and disability from pain appropriately, it is necessary to address both of these areas as separate issues and to assess as well the "psychosocial impact"[60] that the pain problem has on the lives of those individuals who present with pain. The practitioner's failure to do so merely compounds the problem of management and confuses the entire issue. Who is in a better position than the treating physician to assess disability from pain or from some other cause and, further, to assess the psychosocial impact that pain or other disability has on the lives of patients who present with pain, disability, or other impairment (Fig. 1)?

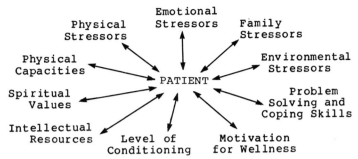

Figure 1. Psychosocial impact of pain.

TREATMENT OF MYOFASCIAL PAIN

The treatment of myofascial pain and dysfunction is dependent on a proper diagnosis, recognizing the specific patterns of referred pain and tenderness and the role of the various perpetuating factors in contributing to the dysfunction seen. Intrinsic mechanical, structural, and postural factors and external static and dynamic forces should be assessed and modified and reconditioning programs instituted, with an emphasis on therapeutic stretching, although therapeutic strengthening should also be part of the treatment program. The major therapeutic goal is to restore balance among the various muscles of the functional (myotatic) unit to achieve normal muscle strength and as full a range of motion as possible. Functional goals, however, should be set at the beginning of a treatment program and modified at periodic intervals thereafter. The use of external supports is recommended, if necessary, to support and protect weak tissues and unstable joints during the course of the reconditioning program, although the practitioner should keep in mind that elastic supports may, if improperly applied, interfere with circulation and in fact set the stage for the development of additional myofascial foci. Goal definition is critical in the early stages of treatment, relative not only to relief of pain but also to what functional outcomes the patient desires, in both the short term and the long term.

The practitioner should always keep in mind that, for the most part, musculoskeletal pain is usually benign disease, and although the psychosocial impact that that disease may have on the patient may be significant, it is the practitioner's responsibility to put the complaints into perspective and to reassure the patient constantly about the benign nature of the presentation. Recurring dysfunction is to be expected as a necessary by-product of performing at as high a level as possible, and when recurring disability occurs, prompt resumption of appropriate treatment should be instituted. Treatment must always be comprehensive, not only paying attention to the apparent physical presentation but also listening for possible subclinical psychosocial distress and "hidden agendas" that may be masquerading as or perpetuating the underlying physical dysfunction. The patient must always be believed, but his dysfunction must always be put into perspective, and his problem-solving and coping skills addressed.

The goal of treatment should always be function oriented, and the impact of pain on the lifestyle of the patient must be critically assessed. Restoration of function must be gradual but progressive. Assessment of the workplace and home environments for physical and emotional stressors, including the necessity to assume prolonged postures for extended periods of time; relationships with family and work associates; and other environmental concerns (temperature, stress, expectations, job satisfaction, and problem resolution), is often critical in achieving an acceptable outcome. Concurrent psychosocial stressors in the home and at work should always be identified and treated with appropriate counseling.

Exercise programs should be moderate but performed on a regular basis, with both therapeutic stretching *and* strengthening on a daily or more frequent basis in a moderate but persistent fashion. Exercises performed for short periods several times a day are preferable to a more intensive session performed once a day. Once motor strength is normal and additional strengthening is desired, the patient can then go into a sports-medicine mode of training, with the subsequent increase in strength and endurance being gradual. The reader should not confuse principles of body building with those of restoring weak muscles to a normal range. Although there is overlap, there are critical differences to keep in mind that are, again, beyond the scope of this article.

Basic exercise should be incorporated into the daily routine and performed moderately throughout the course of the day rather than in one intensive work-out. Patients should be instructed that muscles are the only tissues in the body that have an inherent tendency to get tighter and weaker with disuse, and by incorporating exercise into the activities of daily living or as "tension breakers," recurring disability may be averted. Stretching should be done prior to engaging in more strenuous physical activities and after the performance of those activities. The importance of performing postexercise stretching as part of the cool-down period is often overlooked. If patients have persistent or recurring dysfunction in the work, play, or home environment, it may be appropriate to have them obtain a videotape of themselves "in action" at their work station, in their sport, at home, or in the environment that generally precipitates their dysfunction so that the clinician can detect subtle dysfunctional forces at work. Alternatively, the physician or therapist can make visits to the environment in which the patient lives and works to look for subtle ergonomic dysfunctions.

Medication

The use of medications in the treatment of the myofascial pain syndromes and fibromyalgia is controversial. Although the literature has suggested that anti-inflammatory drugs are no more effective in fibromyalgia than placebo,[29] it has been the author's experience that the use of nonsteroidal anti-inflammatory drugs has been a valuable adjunct, particularly as part of a comprehensive treatment-and-exercise program.[58, 66] Multidisciplinary management appears to be the most effective way for restoring individuals to functional lifestyles.[64, 65] The appropriate use of medications is an integral part of the treatment regimen, and in the author's experience, the use of nonsteroidal anti-inflammatory drugs has been essential, not only in terms of treating the underlying dysfunction but also to assist the patient to be more comfortable as he increases his overall exercise regimen.

Restoration of sleep is essential, and the use of both medications and alternative techniques to facilitate sleep is critical. The use of short-acting hypnotics, along with the longer-acting tricyclics, in low doses has been effective, and once sleep has been restored on a regular basis, gradual tapering of these medications should then be attempted. The use of antihistamines to facilitate sleep has additional benefits in that they also have a direct muscle relaxation effect, and there appears to be an additional benefit in that some patients demonstrate an accelerated histamine release response to palpation and also a "myoedematous response" to injection and palpation (unpublished data).[61] The use of clonidine, in oral or patch form, has recently been recommended by several authors, particularly when there appears to be an active sympathetic-mediated component to the pain, and occasionally, the use of a variety of antianxiety agents, such as alprazolam (Xanax) or diazepam (Valium), may be beneficial, particularly in those patients who present with true tension myalgia, although the clinician should be reminded that the use of the latter medications should be monitored closely because of their tendency to cause dependency and depression.

The use of vitamin C, B complex vitamins, ferrous sulfate, and hormone replacement with thyroid or estrogen, in appropriate individuals, has long been part of the recommended treatment programs, particularly in cases with a slow or poor clinical response or in recurring dysfunction. These agents are all included in the list of perpetuating factors (see Table 2) that must be kept in mind, and corrected, particularly if the clinician is faced with a refractory or recurring clinical problem. The use of vitamin C, in particular, is advised in patients in whom capillary fragility is suspected, and particularly in smokers. It is imperative for patients to discontinue smoking in all cases of refractory pain.[89, 90]

Diagnostic and Therapeutic Injections

Injections are invaluable in both the diagnosis and treatment of myofascial pain and dysfunction. Diagnostically, the injection of lidocaine or procaine into an area of point tenderness can facilitate the search for a local twitch response, which then confirms the diagnosis. Failure to obtain a local twitch response does not mean that a myofascial focus is not present but should prompt a more thorough search for other areas of the muscle or other muscles that may harbor a local twitch response. Similarly, persistent pain or dysfunction following a successful injection should also prompt a search for other trigger points in other areas of the muscle or in other muscles of the myotatic unit, preferably in conjunction with therapeutic stretch-and-spray techniques designed to inactivate all of the trigger points present. The injection of a local anesthetic should immediately abolish the local tenderness and pain and improve strength on manual muscle testing as well as range of motion. The failure to obtain these results after injection serves as a clue that inadequate inactivation of the trigger point has occurred or that the area injected was a tender area rather than a trigger point area. The local injection of an anesthetic can differentiate between local tenderness due to local pathology and referred tenderness from a myofascial focus located elsewhere and can facilitate the finding of the source of that local tenderness much more readily.

From a therapeutic standpoint, injections allow the examiner to inactivate a trigger point rapidly and then perform a more effective therapeutic stretch to the involved muscle group, using a variety of manual medicine techniques to facilitate an effective stretch (muscle energy or contract-relax techniques, ice or cold spray, mobilization, myotherapy, manipulation, myofascial release, and so on). It should be stressed again that an inherent part of the trigger point inactivation process is therapeutic stretching of the muscle treated. Further, after inactivation of the trigger point itself, it is incumbent on the examiner to assess the patient carefully for other satellite trigger points in other parts of the muscle and in other muscles of the functional unit, including the antagonists, the co-movers, and the proximal stabilizers. The use of stretch-and-spray techniques or stretch-and-ice techniques and manual medicine techniques as an adjunct to injection cannot be overemphasized, and the process of injecting a patient without performing any of these ancillary stretching techniques is to be condemned and results merely in long-term therapeutic failure and an alienated patient who will then view the therapeutic injection as short-term relief.

THE GREAT MIMICKER AND POTENTIATOR OF OTHER DISEASES OF THE NEUROMUSCULOSKELETAL SYSTEM

The myofascial pain syndromes can exist independently of other processes, can cause other processes that involve joint or muscle, and can coexist with other processes that involve joint or muscle. They may aggravate or potentiate other coexisting medical conditions involving the neuromusculoskeletal system, and they can mimic other conditions involving the neuromusculoskeletal system.

Many of the entrapment syndromes are caused or aggravated by the concurrent existence of myofascial foci. Apparent static deformities in the various parts of the body can often be reversed by looking for and treating the associated myofascial dysfunction. An awareness of the myofascial syndromes has forced us to reassess our definition of normal range of motion. The myofascial pain syndromes may coexist with other pain states, such as cancer pain, peripheral neuropathy, or arthritic or other rheumatologic process, and may allow the patient to require less narcotics and allow a higher quality of life.

SUMMARY

In summary, this article is designed to give an overview of the role of myofascial pain and dysfunction in treating patients who present with neuromusculoskeletal disability and to convey the fact that we are dealing with an evolving science. Several classifications are suggested to facilitate assessment of the patient who presents with localized or generalized pain and dysfunction. The reader is encouraged to view pain and dysfunction as two separate issues and, further, to think in terms of forces at work causing overload of tissues, as opposed to mere overuse. He or she is encouraged to be global and comprehensive in treatment approaches while, at the same time, focused on the tissue dysfunction seen. Attention must be paid to the physical, emotional, and spiritual values of the patient, as well as the family and work stations in which the patient functions. Patients should always remember that pain involving the musculoskeletal system is usually benign disease, and an integral part of the treatment program involves a return to as functional a lifestyle as possible as quickly as possible, whether pain-free or not. Persistent allegations of disability should be approached from a multidisciplinary standpoint, ensuring that obscure tissue pathology is not overlooked while assisting the patient with problem-solving and coping skills. Return to work or some other functional lifestyle should be gradual and progressive. The hallmarks of treatment include therapeutic stretching and should also include gradual specific strengthening programs, which should be incorporated into the activities of daily living. The use of spray or icing techniques to facilitate stretch, both at home and in the therapeutic environment, should be an integral part of treatment. The use of injections has both diagnostic and therapeutic value, and the use of appropriate medications, with particular emphasis on sleep restoration, and anti-inflammatory drugs has been discussed. The focus of treatment should always be on wellness and on improving problem-solving and coping skills while restoring the individual to a high level of physical conditioning and healthy living. Goal definition at the onset of treatment is imperative to ensure appropriate communication and mutuality of purpose.

References

1. Awad EA: Interstitial myofibrositis: Hypothesis of the mechanism. Arch Phys Med Rehabil 54:449–453, 1973
2. Bach-Andersen R, Jacobsen F, Danneskiold-Samsoe B, et al: New diagnostic tools in primary fibromyalgia. *In* Fricton JR, Awad EA (eds): Myofascial Pain and Fibromyalgia. (Advances in Pain Research and Therapy, vol 17.) New York, Raven Press, 1990
3. Baker BA: The muscle trigger: Evidence of overload injury. Journal of Neurological and Orthopaedic Medicine and Surgery 7:35–43, 1986
4. Bartels EM, Danneskiold-Samsoe B: Histological abnormalities in muscle from patients with certain types of fibrositis. Lancet 1:755–757, 1986
5. Basmajian JV, DeLuca CJ: Muscles Alive: Their Functions as Revealed by Electromyography, ed 5. Baltimore, Williams & Wilkins, 1985
6. Beeson PB, McDermott W (eds): Cecil-Loeb Textbook of Medicine ed 11. Philadelphia, WB Saunders, 1963
7. Bengtsson A, Henriksson K-G, Jorfeldt L, et al: Primary fibromyalgia, a clinical and laboratory study of 55 patients. Scand J Rheumatol 15:340–347, 1986
8. Bengtsson A, Henriksson K-G, Larsson J: Reduced high-energy phosphate levels in painful muscles in patients with primary fibromyalgia. Arthritis Rheum 29:817–821, 1986
9. Bengtsson A, Henriksson K-G, Larsson J: Muscle biopsy in primary fibromyalgia. Scand J Rheumatol 15:1–6, 1986
10. Bennett RM: Fibrositis-fibromyalgia syndrome. *In* Schumacher HR (ed): Primer on Rheumatic Diseases, ed 9. Atlanta, Arthritis Foundation, 1988
11. Bennett RM (ed): Fibrositis/fibromyalgia syndrome: Current issues and perspectives. Am J Med 81(3A), 1986
12. Bennett RM: Fibrositis: Misnomer for a common rheumatic disorder. West J Med 134:405–413, 1981
13. Caro XJ: Immunofluorescent detection of IgG at the dermal-epidermal junction in patients with apparent primary fibrositis syndrome. Arthritis Rheum 27:1174–1179, 1984
14. Cyriax J: Textbook of Orthopaedic Medicine, ed 5, vol 1. Baltimore, Williams & Wilkins, 1969
15. Cyriax J: Textbook of Orthopaedic Medicine, vol 2. Philadelphia, Baillière Tindall, 1984
16. Dexter JR, Simons DG: Local twitch response in human muscle evoked by palpation and needle penetration of a trigger point. Arch Phys Med Rehabil 62:521, 1981
17. Enestrom S, Bengtsson A, Lindstrom F, et al: Attachment of IgG to dermal extracellular matrix in patients with fibromyalgia. Clin Exp Rheumatol 8(2):127–135, 1990
18. Escobar PL, Ballesteros J: Myofascial pain syndrome. Ortho Rev 16:708, 1987
19. Fields HL: Pain from deep tissues and referred pain. *In* Pain. New York, McGraw-Hill, 1987
20. Fischer AA: Pressure tolerance over muscles and bones in normal subjects. Arch Phys Med Rehabil 67:406–409, 1986
21. Fischer AA: Pressure threshold meter: Its use for quantification of tender spots. Arch Phys Med Rehabil 67:836–838, 1986
22. Fischer AA: Documentation of myofascial trigger points. Arch Phys Med Rehabil 16:286, 1988
23. Fischer AA: Application of pressure algometry in manual medicine. Journal of Manual Medicine 5:145–150, 1990
24. Fischer AA: Differential diagnosis of muscle tenderness and pain. Pain Management Jan/Feb 1991, pp 30–36
25. Fricton JR: Myofascial pain syndromes. *In* Fricton JR, Awad EA (eds): Myofascial Pain and Fibromyalgia. (Advances in Pain Research and Therapy, vol 17.) New York, Raven Press, 1990
26. Fricton JR, Awad EA (eds): Myofascial Pain and Fibromyalgia. (Advances in Pain Research and Therapy, vol 17.) New York, Raven Press, 1990
27. Fricton JR, Auvinen MD, Dykstra D, et al: Myofascial pain syndrome: Electromyo-

graphic changes associated with local twitch response. Arch Phys Med Rehabil 66:314–317, 1984
28. Fry HJH: Prevalence of overuse (injury) syndrome in Australian music schools. Br J Ind Med 44:35–40, 1987
29. Goldenberg DL, Felson DT, Dinerman H: Randomized control trial of amitriptyline and naproxen in the treatment of patients with fibromyalgia. Arthritis Rheum 29:1371–1377, 1986
30. Goldenberg DL, Simms RW, Geiger A, et al: High frequency of fibromyalgia in patients with chronic fatigue seen in a primary care practice. Arthritis Rheum 33:381–387, 1990
31. Gowers WR: Lumbago: Its lessons in analogues. Br Med J 1:117–121, 1904
32. Greenman PE: Principles of Manual Medicine. Baltimore, Williams & Wilkins, 1989
33. Headley BJ: EMG and myofascial pain. Clinical Management 10(4):43–46, 1990
34. Hench PS: The problem of rheumatism and arthritis. Ann Intern Med 10:880, 1936
35. Henriksson K-G, Bengtsson A: Muscular changes in fibromyalgia and their significance in diagnosis. In Fricton JR, Awad EA (eds): Myofascial Pain and Fibromyalgia. (Advances in Pain Research and Therapy, vol. 17.) New York, Raven Press, 1990
36. Hong C-Z, Simons DG, Statham L: Electromyographic analysis of local twitch responses of human extensor digitorum communis muscle during ischemic compression over the arm. Arch Phys Med Rehabil 67:680, 1986
37. Kellgren JH: A preliminary account of referred pains arising from muscle. Br Med J 1:325, 1938
38. Kellgren JH: On the distribution of pain arising from deep somatic structures with charts of segmental pain areas. Clin Sci 4:35, 1939
39. Klein I, Parker M, Shebert R, et al: Hypothyroidism presenting as muscle stiffness and pseudohypertrophy: Hoffman's syndrome. Am J Med 70:891, 1981
40. Kraft GH, Johnson EW, LaBan MM: The fibrositis syndrome. Arch Phys Med Rehabil 49:155, 1968
41. Kraus H, Fischer AA: Diagnosis and treatment of myofascial pain. Mt Sinai J Med 58:3, 1991
42. Krejci V, Koch P: Muscle and Tendon Injuries in Athletes. Chicago, Year Book, 1979
43. Lewis T, Kellgren JH: Observations relating to referral pain, visceromotor reflexes and other associated phenomena. Clin Sci 4:47, 1939
44. Lewit K: The needle effect in the relief of myofascial pain. Pain 6:83–90, 1979
45. Lewit K: Postisometric relaxation in combination with other methods of muscular facilitation and inhibition. Manual Medicine 2:101–104, 1986
46. Lewit K, Simons DG: Myofascial pain: Relief by post-isometric relaxation. Arch Phys Med Rehabil 65:452–456, 1984
47. Maitland GD: Peripheral Manipulation, ed 2. London, Butterworths, 1977
48. Melzack R: Myofascial trigger points: Relation to acupuncture and mechanisms of pain. Arch Phys Med Rehabil 62:114, 1981
49. Mense S: Physiology of nociception in muscles. In Fricton JR, Awad EA (eds): Myofascial Pain and Fibromyalgia. (Advances in Pain Research and Therapy, vol 17). New York, Raven Press, 1990
50. Moldofsky H: The contribution of sleep-wave physiology to fibromyalgia. In Fricton JR, Awad EA (eds): Myofascial Pain and Fibromyalgia. (Advances in Pain Research and Therapy, vol 17.) New York, Raven Press, 1990
51. Moldofsky H, Tullis C, Lue FA: Sleep related myoclonus and rheumatic pain modulation disorder (fibrositis syndrome). J Rheumatol 13:614–617, 1986
52. Pellegrino MJ, Waylonis GW, Sommer A: Familial occurrence of primary fibromyalgia. Arch Phys Med Rehabil 70:61–63, 1989
53. Raj PP: Practical Management of Pain. Chicago, Year Book, 1986
54. Retzlaff EW, Berry AH, Haight AS, et al: The piriformis muscle syndrome. J Am Osteopath Assoc 73:799, 1974
55. Reynolds MD: Myofascial trigger point syndromes in the practice of rheumatology. Arch Phys Med Rehabil 62:111–114, 1981
56. Rogers EJ, Rogers R: Fibromyalgia and myofascial pain, either, neither, or both? Orthop Rev 18:1217, 1989

57. Rosen NB: Myofascial pain—a means for more effective communication with the dysfunctional patient with pain. Presented at the Annual Meetings of the American Academy of Physical Medicine and Rehabilitation, Boston, MA, October 1984

58. Rosen NB: Treating the many facets of pain. Business and Health 3(May):6, 7–10, 1986

59. Rosen NB: Myofascial pain: the hidden disease of the athlete. Presented at the 1987 Meeting of the North American Academy of Manipulation Medicine, Las Vegas, NV, 1987

60. Rosen NB: Seminar on Perpetuating factors in myofascial pain: Wellness and illness behavior as perpetuating factors in pain management. Presented at the Annual Meetings of the American Academy of Physical Medicine and Rehabilitation, Orlando, FL, October 1987

61. Rosen NB: Seminar on advances in the diagnosis and management of myofascial pain syndromes: A critical look at the spectrum of "fibrositis." Presented at the Annual Meetings of the American Academy of Physical Medicine and Rehabilitation, Phoenix, AZ, October 1990

62. Rosen NB: Seminar on focal myofascial pain disorders: An overview of the focal myofascial pain disorders. Presented at the Annual Meetings of the American Academy of Physical Medicine and Rehabilitation, Washington, DC, October 1991

63. Rosen NB: Myofascial pain: The great mimicker and potentiator of other diseases in musicians. Presented at the Performing Arts Symposium, Medical and Chirurgical Faculty of the State of Maryland, January 1992

64. Rosen NB, Sharoff KA: Return to work: Criteria for success or failure of a pain treatment program. Presented at the Annual Meetings of the American Academy of Physical Medicine and Rehabilitation, Boston, MA, October 1984

65. Rosen NB, Sharoff KA: Role of selective hospitalization in returning the patient to work. Presented at the Annual Meetings of the American Academy of Physical Medicine and Rehabilitation, Boston, MA, October 1984

66. Rosen NB, Sharoff KA, Khanna VK: The dysfunctional pain patient—returning to work: A preliminary report. Md Med J 34:605–608, 1985

67. Rubin D: Myofascial trigger point syndromes: An approach to management. Arch Phys Med Rehabil 62:107, 1981

68. Russell IJ: Neurohormonal aspects of fibromyalgia syndrome. Rheum Dis Clin North Am 15:149, 1989

69. Scudds RA, Trachsel LC, Luckhurst BJ, et al: A comparative study of pain, sleep quality and pain responsiveness in fibrositis and myofascial pain syndrome. J Rheumatol Suppl 19:120, 1989

70. Sessle BJ: Central nervous system mechanisms of muscular pain. In Fricton JR, Awad EA (eds): Myofascial Pain and Fibromyalgia. (Advances in Pain Research and Therapy, vol 17.) Raven Press, New York, 1990

71. Shulman LE, Bumin JJ: Disorders of the joints. In Harrison TR (ed): Principles of Internal Medicine, ed 3. New York, McGraw-Hill, Inc, 1958

72. Simons DG: Muscle pain syndromes. 1. Am J Phys Med 54:289–311, 1975

73. Simons DG: Muscle pain syndromes. 2. Am J Phys Med 55:15–42, 1976

74. Simons DG: Myofascial pain syndromes due to trigger points. 1. Principles, diagnosis, and perpetuating factors. Manual Medicine 1:67–71, 1985

75. Simons DG: Myofascial pain syndromes due to trigger points. 2. Treatment and single-muscle syndromes. Manual Medicine 1:72–77, 1985

76. Simons DG: Fibrositis/fibromyalgia: A form of myofascial trigger points? Am J Med 81 (suppl 3A):93–98, 1986

77. Simons DG: Myofascial pain syndromes due to trigger points. In Goodgold J (ed): Rehabilitation Medicine. St Louis, CV Mosby, 1988

78. Simons DG: Muscular pain syndromes. In Fricton JR, Awad EA (eds): Myofascial Pain and Fibromyalgia. (Advances in Pain Research and Therapy, vol 17.) New York, Raven Press, 1990

79. Simons DG, Travell JG: Myofascial origins of low back pain. 1. Principles of diagnosis and treatment. Postgrad Med 73:66–77, 1983

80. Simons DG, Travell JG: Myofascial origins of low back pain. 2. Torso muscles. Postgrad Med 73:81–92, 1983

81. Simons DG, Travell JG: Myofascial origins of low back pain. 3. Pelvic and lower extremity muscles. Postgrad Med 73:99–108, 1983
82. Skootsky SA, Jaeger B, Oye RK: Prevalence of myofascial pain in general internal medicine practice. West J Med 151:157–160, 1989
83. Smythe HA: Tender points: Evolution of concepts of the fibrositis/fibromyalgia syndrome. Am J Med 81(3A):2–6, 1986
84. Smythe HA, Moldofsky H: Two contributions to understanding of the "fibrositis" syndrome. Bull Rheum Dis 28:928–931, 1977
85. Thompson JM: Tension myalgia as a diagnosis at the Mayo Clinic and its relationship to fibrositis, fibromyalgia and myofascial pain syndromes. Mayo Clin Proc 65:1237–1248, 1990
86. Travell JG: Chronic myofascial pain syndromes: Mysteries of the history. In Fricton JR, Awad EA (eds): Myofascial Pain and Fibromyalgia. (Advances in Pain Research and Therapy, vol 17.) New York, Raven Press, 1990
87. Travell JG, Daitz B: Myofascial Pain Syndromes: The Travell Trigger-Point Tapes. Baltimore, Williams & Wilkins, 1990
88. Travell J, Rinzler SH: The myofascial genesis of pain. Postgrad Med 11:425–434, 1952
89. Travell JG, Simons DG: Myofascial Pain and Dysfunction: The Trigger Point Manual. Baltimore, Williams & Wilkins, 1983
90. Travell JG, Simons DG: Myofascial Pain and Dysfunction: The Trigger Point Manual, vol II. Baltimore, Williams & Wilkins, 1991
91. Wallace DJ, Peter JD, et al: Fibromyalgia, cytokines, fatigue syndromes, and immune regulation. In Fricton JR, Awad EA (eds): Myofascial Pain and Fibromyalgia. (Advances in Pain Research and Therapy, vol 17.) New York, Raven Press, 1990
92. Williams PC: Pain in the back. In Harrison TR (ed): Principles of Internal Med, ed 3. New York, McGraw-Hill, 1958
93. Wolfe F: The clinical syndrome of fibrositis. Am J Med 81(3A):7–14, 1986
94. Wolfe F: Fibrositis, fibromyositis, and musculoskeletal disease: The current status of the fibrositis syndrome. Arch Phys Med Rehabil 69:527, 1988
95. Wolfe F: Two muscle pain syndromes: Fibromyalgia and the myofascial pain syndrome. Pain Management 3:153–164, 1990
96. Wolfe F, Hawley D, Cathey MA, et al: Fibrositis: Symptom frequency and criteria for diagnosis. J Rheumatol 12:1159–1163, 1985
97. Wolfe F, Smythe HA, Yunus MB, et al: Multicenter Fibromyalgia Criteria Committee. Arthritis Rheum 32 (suppl 4):S47, 1989
98. Wolfe F, Smythe HA, Yunus MB, et al: American College of Rheumatology 1990 criteria for the classification of fibromyalgia: Report of the Multicenter Criteria Committee. Arthritis Rheum 33:160–172, 1990
99. Wyngaarden JB, Smith LA (eds): Cecil Textbook of Medicine, ed 17. Philadelphia, WB Saunders, 1985
100. Young RR, Bradley WG, Adams RD: Diseases of striated muscle. In Petersdorf RG (ed): Harrison's Principles of Internal Medicine, ed 10. New York, McGraw-Hill, 1983
101. Yunus M, Masi AT, Calabro JJ, et al: Primary fibromyalgia (fibrositis): Clinical study of 50 patients with matched normal controls. Semin Arthritis Rheum 11:151–171, 1981
102. Yunus M, Masi AT, Calabro JJ, et al: Primary fibromyalgia. Am Fam Physician 25:115–121, 1982

Address reprint requests to

Norman B. Rosen, MD
129 Beech Bark Lane
Baltimore, MD 21204

LEGAL ISSUES INVOLVED IN THE OUTPATIENT MANAGEMENT OF PAIN

Jay Meythaler, JD, MD

Whether we like it or not, we live in a litigious society. Dealing with legal issues is a part of any medical practice that involves treating patients with pain, because the pain is often claimed to be disabling and frequently is the result of injuries at work or in an accident. The result may be compensated or uncompensated time-off, partial disability, or full disability. Because of the financial issues involved, society has placed on physicians an obligation to become knowledgeable about those areas of the law that involve us. We, as physicians, need to become involved to enable our patients to obtain the necessary medical services they deserve. At the same time we need to ensure that the accepted standards of care are not breached, because this may result in filing of a lawsuit. Additionally, strict adherence to standards will improve physician reimbursement for any care provided.

So how can we physicians fulfill our roles with regard to supplying proper and useful information to various agencies such as the Social Security Administration, worker's compensation boards, the judiciary, or to other lawyers in third party lawsuits? Proper documentation is necessary for physicians to ensure their patients get the medical care they deserve and are not placed in a situation that may result in reinjury or further disability. If one is involved in pain management, it is inevitable that someone will attempt to have you testify as an expert witness. On the other side, one needs to avoid the accusation of not following the general accepted standards of care, which may result in a malpractice suit. Finally, to survive as professionals we need to ensure proper documentation of what has been provided in the way of services for our patients for appropriate reimbursement. I address each of these issues herein.

From Spain Rehabilitation Center, Department of Rehabilitation Medicine, University of Alabama School of Medicine, Birmingham, Alabama

PHYSICAL MEDICINE AND REHABILITATION CLINICS OF NORTH AMERICA

DETERMINATION OF DISABILITY

Workers' Compensation

In most states, physicians have a legal obligation to supply appropriate information when treating workers who are covered by workers' compensation insurance.[21] There is nearly universal agreement that the quality and timeliness of reporting have a great effect on the cost of care. The information the physician is obligated to provide includes the following:

Date of injury
Circumstances surrounding the injury
Pertinent objective physical findings in laboratory data
Diagnosis
Planned treatment or further treatment required
Recommended activity level, including such things as lifting (including weight restrictions); amount of walking, standing, stooping, twisting, turning, and repetitive hand motions; and, finally, use of special equipment such as ladders
Prognosis for further recovery, if any
Impairment or disability rating
Any additional pertinent information, particularly circumstances that may affect the outcome—one that is well known is whether there is a planned lawsuit on the horizon.

Formerly, it was considered proper to consider only objective criteria in developing the disability rating; however, most state laws are framed within the context of the disability's effect on the specific occupational task. It has been interpreted by some that the physician has a responsibility to present an opinion on this issue, even though it is based in part on subjective criteria.[13] One of the most complex issues with regard to disability is the effect of pain on disability. Ignoring pain in the impairment rating is not a solution to the problem. Despite its subjectiveness, most physicians know that pain contributes to the overall disability.[17, 19] Indeed, some courts recognize the right of the expert to take into account the effect that pain may have on a patient's disability.[19] Although administrators or judges determine the disability, the physician's opinion, including the effect that pain may have on the amount of disability, can influence the final outcome. This is important because, in times of tight budgets, it is easy for the administrators to convert the objective impairments scale to a final disability rating without considering the effect of pain on the individual's capacity to perform his or her occupational role. There are usually a number of objective criteria found in each state's workers' compensation law; however, state standards may vary in how they both set impairment ratings and assess disability, but certain definitions are fairly universal.

Impairment refers to an anatomic or physiologic defect that impairs an individual's ability to perform certain functions in a standard fashion. This results in a restriction in the ability of an individual to perform this function (a functional limitation). Even though the person may still be able to perform the task with modifications, there is a functional limitation due to the impairment. In addition to the various state-mandated systems, there are two other universal impairment rating systems that can be used when the state systems do not have specific guidelines to define impairment. The most common is the American Medical Association's *Guide to the Evaluation of Permanent Impairment.*[5] The other is the

American Academy of Orthopaedic Surgeons' *Manual for Orthopaedic Surgeons in Evaluating Permanent Physical Impairment.*[4] Disability is defined as the interaction between the individual and the environment. It encompasses not only the medical impairment but also the motivation, educational level, work experience, emotional and psychological factors, age, socioeconomic background, and financial status of the individual involved. Many states have a preset reimbursement depending on the amount or percentage of disability.[19]

Social Security Disability

The largest disability insurance program in the world is the US Social Security Administration. The system is based on an insurance model of work disability and is funded through the payroll taxes of the workers. It is an earned right of all workers (Title II) who have worked for approximately 5 of the past 10 years, have a current income of less than $300 per month, and have been unemployed for the previous 6 months.[12] Under the Supplemental Security Income Program (Title XVI), it can be awarded to the needy, aged, blind, and disabled if they qualify under specific financial need qualifications.[12] The Social Security Administration's test of disability is that an individual should be unable "to engage in any substantial gainful activity by reason of any medically determinable physical or mental impairment which can be expected to result in death, or which has lasted or can be expected to last for a continuous period of less than twelve months."[12] In this system, the physician is expected to comment only on the individual's medical impairment and is not expected to comment on the disability or employability.[8] Rather, the Social Security Administration is specifically instructed to downplay such comments if they are offered.[6, 24] It is not until the individual is well along the appeals process, when he or she is in front of the administrative law judge, that medical opinion is permissible, welcomed, and often persuasive. Indeed, it is in the individual's interest to appeal because as many as 50% of cases appealed to the administrative law judge level are reversed in favor of the applicant (Fig. 1).[8] This is when expert medical testimony may be quite useful.

TESTIFYING

One cannot avoid becoming an expert witness if one is involved in workers' compensation issues, Social Security Administration matters, or third-party lawsuits. An *expert witness* is an individual with technical expertise in the area under consideration. The common law in the United States holds that a jury, which is generally composed of laymen, does not generally have the sufficient technical expertise to render judgment on technical issues, such as medicine, without the input of experts. The purpose of the expert witness is to provide information that the jurors or judge ordinarily would not have on their own. Only in the most flagrantly negligent cases is an expert witness not required.[6] The expert's functions in court are to establish the standard of care for the specialty involved and to aid in the determination of damages. Because physicians in physical medicine and rehabilitation are rarely sued, the standard-of-care issue arises quite infrequently. More important, particularly in pain management, is the involvement of damages. In this area one can hardly avoid becoming involved, because the specialty is concerned with returning the individual to as functional a life as possible.

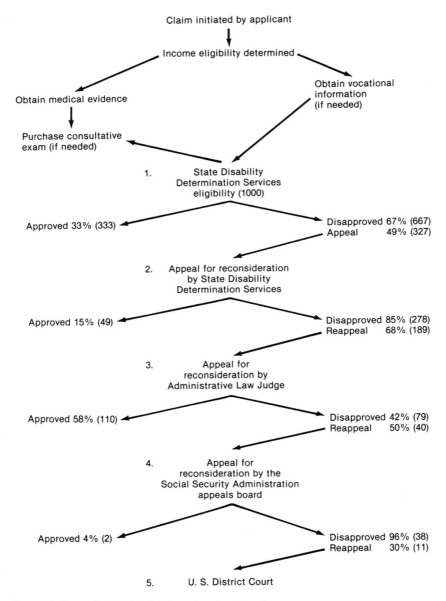

Figure 1. Steps in the Social Security disability insurance application and appeals process. A total of 495 of 1000 applications (49.5%) are approved. Number in parentheses corresponds to 1000 initial applicants. (*From* Carey TS, Hadler NM: The role of the primary physician in disability determination for Social Security insurance and workers' compensation. Ann Intern Med 104:706–710, 1986; with permission.)

The issues a physician should be ready to address in court are the following:

Since the time of the injury or illness in question, has the patient's medical care been appropriate and reasonable in cost?
Has the patient more potential for recovery?
Is there more medical treatment required in the future?
What is the possibility of new or developing medical complications as a result of the illness or injury, and what are the potential costs of this medical care?

In some situations you will be asked what kind or kinds of occupations would the individual involved be physically capable of performing in the future. This is done so that one can then estimate the lost earning capacity of the individual for damages. Also, sometimes you will be asked whether any special requirements, such as equipment and personnel, will be required for the person to live reasonably. These issues are usually addressed in life care plans, which are compiled by economists and consultants of the plaintiff's legal staff, and you are frequently asked to review them. Along the same lines, vocational counselors are asked about the costs and nature of vocational and educational training, and psychologists are often asked about emotional and psychological impairments. Because you are the leader of the rehabilitation team, they may ask your opinion of their opinions.

Why should one become involved as an expert witness? The most obvious reason is so that your patient or the individual involved obtains the necessary services, both medical and otherwise, for him or her to be able to return to as functional, productive, and rewarding a life as possible. The reality is that there are always experts who testify for the other side (the so-called hired guns), and it is the responsibility of every physician to ensure that justice is done. Otherwise, despite our legal system's shortcomings, you have no right to complain about the outrageous awards recently made by the legal system. Ignoring the problem does not make it go away, and it certainly does not do the patients any good, either. Just as frequently, patients do not receive the medical services, equipment, and personnel they need to live reasonably.

What are the elements of being an expert witness, and how should you approach the problem? Can you be subpoenaed as an expert witness? You must realize that you will be subpoenaed; however, a subpoena can require one only to give objective evidence or to bring certain materials, such as medical records. One cannot be forced to be an expert witness, but after you "volunteer" to be an expert witness, you usually will be subpoenaed to ensure that you will appear at the agreed time and bring any record or other objective material on which you have based your opinion to the hearing or deposition. When you get involved, be sure to draw up a letter of agreement with the attorney who has asked you to cooperate with him. Medicine is a service industry, and "time is money." An excellent letter has been presented as an example (Fig. 2).[10]

Once in court or in a deposition, there are various techniques of testifying. First, what is the definition of a specialist in your area, such as physical medicine and rehabilitation? This is required from you in almost every deposition and trial in which you become involved. The one that I use most frequently is that "physical medicine and rehabilitation is a specialty of medicine primarily concerned with 'the development of a person to the fullest physical, psychological, social, vocational, avocational, and educational potential consistent with his or her physiological or anatomical impairment and environmental limitations.'[11] Physicians in physical medicine and rehabilitation deal with patients who have

Dear Attorney:

I've received your subpoena (or request for medical report or records) concerning (_____).

Naturally, I'll be happy to assist you. My fee for a brief medical report is $_____. (That's extra work for me, and my meter is running.) This will include full details of the incident in question, my full diagnosis, and the best prognosis I can give, including my impressions of the patient's degree of disability.

If you wish, I'll fully review this patient's records regarding other factors that may relate to this case for $_____. (It might be helpful if you knew that the patient had back trouble and was impotent seven years prior to the accident, but I'm not going to spend a hour going through his chart unless you pay me for my time.)

My fee for serving as an expert medical witness is $_____ an hour. It is not, of course, contingent on the outcome of the case. (If I cancel a day's appointments for your case, I expect to get paid--win, lose, or settle.) I charge a two-hour minimum to review the case and pertinent records before trial, and a four-hour minimum if the case is scheduled but not heard.

I strongly advise a pretrial conference to review the medical evidence and my testimony. We can do this at my office at my hourly rate, or at your office at my half-day rate.

I must ask for payment in advance for all medical reports, and all other charges will be due as they occur. (If you can persuade my creditors to wait for me to pay them until you've paid me, I'll give you all the free credit you want. Otherwise, pay up front.)

Since we haven't worked together before, I'm enclosing a copy of my curriculum vitae. It documents specific continuing education courses of this type.

If you feel that this case will likely go to trial, we'll need to arrange for anatomical models or visual aids to help the jurors. I'll have the patient's X-ray, but they'll be useless in court without a view box.

I realize that you aren't now able to specify the exact day of my testimony. My secretary has my vacation and meeting schedule for the next three months. Your client probably would be unhappy about paying for me to fly back from a meeting to testify, and while I try to be objective, a last-minute change of vacation plans isn't likely to put me in the best frame of mind toward you and your client.

As soon as the case is scheduled, please notify my secretary.

Yours truly,

Charles Davant III, M.D.

Figure 2. A medical-expert letter. (*From* Davant C: Short-notice subpoenas don't bother me anymore. Medical Economics, May 7, 1990; with permission. Copyright © 1990 by Medical Economics Publishing Company.)

suffered primarily, although not exclusively, muscular, skeletal, or neurologic pathology." I have used this definition frequently, and it appears to satisfy both juries and judges.

When you go to court, in most cases, you are allowed to take notes with you to the stand or deposition, and you are free to refer to them; however, you must remember that they can be entered into the official record and reviewed by the opposing attorney. Consequently, it is best that you review with the attorney who has requested you to be an expert witness the notes you will take to the stand, so they cannot be used in a misleading or confusing manner. You should always have with you an updated curriculum vitae to make available to the court. It is often used as an aid in establishing you as an expert in the area in which you are testifying.

LEGAL LIABILITY

Avoiding a Malpractice Suit

The first thing to realize is that physical medicine and rehabilitation specialists dealing with pain patients in an outpatient practice are not in a specialty with high risk for being sued. This is not to say that you can never be sued. The first way to avoid being sued is to talk to your patients. It has been clearly established that those physicians who talk to their patients are more likely to avoid being sued. Being accused of negligence is by far the cause of most medical malpractice suits[6]; however, there are other causes, such as lack of informed consent or even contractual arrangements.

Lawsuits for any shortcomings in the delivery of medical care and for aspects that are not specifically agreed on (contractual arrangements) are covered by an area of the law called *torts*. Under tort law, an individual owes a duty to others to avoid causing them injury and to act as a "reasonable person." The general duty a doctor owes to a patient whom he has agreed to treat is to exercise the degree of knowledge and skill normally possessed under similar circumstances by other doctors and to use ordinary and reasonable care in the treatment of the patient.[6] As a general rule, the law imposes no duty on any person, including physicians, to assist in the preservation of a person's life or health.[18] This is based on a prevalent legal theory on which legal liability for medical care is based, the contract model of medical care. In the contract model of medical care, a contract is voluntarily entered into by both parties, the physician and the patient.[20, 26] It imposes a fiduciary obligation of the physician to act in the patient's interest and to provide the patient with a standard of competent medical care. Voluntariness is preserved for both parties in this system. The patient can leave the physician at any time. Similarly, the physician is free to sever the relationship, provided that the patient is given sufficient opportunity to find another physician. The contract model allows the physician virtually complete freedom in choosing to enter into a treatment contract with the patient; however, once he or she has agreed to treat the patient, there are certain obligations. To be sued for malpractice, it must be established legally that there was negligence by the physician in not fulfilling his obligations. The plaintiff must prove four elements to establish negligence.

> The physician had a duty to the patient to conform to a specific standard of care.
> The physician breached that duty.

The physician's breach was the actual and approximate cause of the patient's injury.

The patient suffered damage from that breach of duty or obligation.

The standard of care is not intended to make the physician ensure the success of his diagnosis and treatment, nor does it require the physician to provide the highest degree of care known to his profession.[7]

To determine whether the aforementioned four elements have been met, the jury may rely on one of three methods of evaluation. The first is expert witness testimony, covered earlier. The purpose of the expert witness, as stated previously, is to provide information that the jurors or judge ordinarily would not have on their own. In most medical cases, expert testimony is required to establish negligence.[6, 9] Experts are not called on to give an opinion about whether a particular physician has been negligent. Rather, an expert witness may provide an opinion about a theoretical situation, which is always presented as being very similar to the facts of the case before the court[6]; however, there is another method of evaluation called the *common knowledge experience*.[6] When the situation is so obvious as to be apparent to a layperson or is within the common knowledge of a layperson, expert testimony is not required.[23] This happens, for example, when a physician fails to attend to a patient under his care, with obvious and potentially serious complications.[23] The final method of evaluation is the legal theory of *res ipsa loquitur*. This term is Latin for "the thing speaks for itself." Theory has long been used in the common law to prove those things that could not, by witness report, be proven. It was first applied in a case in California and has been infrequently used since then.[25] To use the doctrine, three elements must be met:

The accident must be of a kind that would not ordinarily have occurred in the absence of someone's negligence.

The accident must be caused by something or someone under the exclusive control of the person accused.

The accident must not be due either to a voluntary action or to the contributory negligence of the person injured.

The legal doctrine of *res ipsa loquitur* is used when it is reasonably clear that something has gone wrong during an operation or procedure that was under the physician's control and from which the plaintiff suffers harm.[22] This is significant because, under this doctrine, the burden of proof is shifted onto the physician to show that there was no negligence.[22]

Informed Consent

Another cause for being sued is "lack of informed consent." This issue has been linked to a great increase in the number of lawsuits filed in the past 10 to 15 years.[15] All patients have the right to accept or decline medical treatment, based on their individual assessment of the risks and benefits of the proposed treatment and the alternatives available. Under the doctrine of informed consent, a physician has the duty to advise the patient of the nature of the proposed treatment, its inherent risks, and the alternatives of such a treatment, as well as the probability of success. Informed consent can only be forgone in a medical emergency.[1, 2]

Contractual Obligations

Under the contractual model of care, another cause for a legal suit is lack of provision of continuing care after the physician institutes treatment. One can be sued for refusing to see the patient, under the doctrine of abandonment, unless the patient is transferred to another appropriate setting and another physician institutes care.[2, 3] Of course, refusing to see the patient would have to result in damages for there to be any monetary recovery. The only other contractual method of being sued is for the physician to guarantee or warrant outcomes.[14]

Strict Liability

Recently, there has been a significant amount of discussion in the medical literature about the trend towards "strict liability." In strict liability, a physician could be held liable for any adverse outcomes, regardless of fault. This has been advanced recently to explain the increase in claim frequency and awards; however, there appears to be little evidence that the common law standard of liability has changed.[15] It has been suggested this is more likely a result of increased specialization within the legal community, permitting a larger capital investment in malpractice cases, an increased sharing of knowledge, an increased number of legal specialists, and better preparation for litigation.[15] It is still estimated by the legal society that there are many more cases of malpractice that are never filed than are awarded.[15]

In the outpatient setting of pain management, I believe the most frequent causes of legal suits against physicians occur

- in the use of procedures such as epidural injections, particularly when there is no informed consent
- in missing a more significant injury, such as an unstable fracture, before prescribing therapy or exercises
- in the improper use of medications, particularly in not checking for previous allergies or adverse reactions in the patient.

Billing

To avoid being accused of fraudulently billing for services that were not provided, services that you have provided as a physician should be documented properly. This issue is taking more and more of our time as physicians but is required if one is to avoid being accused of fraudulently billing for services that were not provided. This is a very important issue in Medicare and Medicaid. It has not been helped by the increase of confusion since the implementation of the resource-based relative value system; however, if one takes the proper time to document and uses some general common sense, significant problems in this area can usually be avoided. The problem is time, and "time is money" in a service profession. One aid in reimbursement is to document the amount of time needed beyond what would be expected, such as for patient counseling and education. Another is to divide written or dictated notes clearly into sections of history, physical examination, impressions, and so one, which makes it easier for the reviewers to scan for the various elements that they are looking for when reviewing the level of service billed for. For a comprehensive disability evaluation, I include the following elements:

1. Chief complaint
2. History of present illness, including the following:
   a. Name of employer
   b. Account of illness, including onset and specific episodes
   c. Specific treatment one has received, including hospitalizations, medications, therapy, and prescribed physical restrictions
3. Past medical history, including any previous conditions that may affect this illness or injury
4. Family medical history
5. Social history, including education
6. Work history, which should include the job title, description of the position, physical requirements, income, and dates for all previously held positions as well as the current position
7. Physical examination
8. Medical impression, including the following:
   a. Summary of objective findings supporting the diagnosis, impairments, or functional limitations
   b. Description of impairments, including any percentages assigned and the reference used to determine the percentage of the body part or total body
   c. Description of functional limitations, with specific activity restrictions
   d. Relation of the functional limitations to work, including the activity restrictions, dates off work, and further job possibilities or limits
   e. Causal relation of the injury or illness to the disability
9. Recommendations, including:
   a. Further treatment suggested, including further activity levels, equipment, and environmental modifications required, as well as future medical needs
   b. Expected future course of the illness or injury with or without treatment
   c. Percentage of disability

It must also be ensured that there is reimbursement for the ancillary outpatient services provided at your hospital or clinic. This is particularly important if the physician wants to continue having privileges in that institution. Most of these requirements are spelled out by the accreditating organizations.[16] The physician should include in his or her orders to therapists the pertinent diagnosis; the specified treatment, including the goals of treatment; any precautions of which to be aware; and when the patient's progress will be reevaluted.

CONCLUSION

In the medical practice of pain management, involvement with legal issues is unavoidable. The physician must consider it a part of his or her medical practice. Proper documentation saves considerable time and headaches down the road. Because "time is money," one should not be afraid to bill for expertise when one's opinion is requested. Becoming educated regarding the legal process improves the efficiency of one's practice and facilitates the medical care of patients.

References

1. 61 Am. Jur. 2d Physicians, Surgeons, etc. 160, 1981
2. 61 Am. Jur. 2d Physicians, Surgeons, etc. 234, 1981
3. 61 Am. Jur. 2d Physicians, Surgeons, etc. 236–239, 1981

 4. American Academy of Orthopaedic Surgeons: Manual for Orthopaedic Surgeons in Evaluating Permanent Physical Impairment. Chicago, American Academy of Orthopaedic Surgeons, 1962
 5. American Medical Association: Guides to the Evaluation of Permanent Impairment, ed 2. Chicago, American Medical Association, 1984
 6. Becker VV: Medical negligence: The duty. Contemp Orthop 20:125–128, 1990
 7. Brown v. Kaulizaskis, 229 Va. 524, 331 S.E.2d 440 (1985)
 8. Carey TS, Hadler NM: The role of the primary physician in disability determination for Social Security insurance and worker's compensation. Ann Intern Med 104:706–710, 1986
 9. Collins v. Meeker, 424 P2d 488 (Kansas, 1967)
10. Davant C: Short term subpoenas don't bother me anymore. Medical Economics, May 7, 1990, pp 120–125
11. Delisa JA, Martin GM, Currie DM: Rehabilitation medicine: Past, present, and future. *In* Delisa JA (ed): Rehabilitation Medicine. Philadelphia, JB Lippincott, 1988, pp 3–24
12. Disability Evaluation Under Social Security: A Handbook for Physicians. Washington, DC, U.S. Department of Health, Education and Welfare, 1979
13. Dobyns JH: Role of the physician in worker's compensation injuries. J Hand Surg [Am] 12:826–829, 1987
14. Hawkins v. McGee, 146 A. 641 (New Hampshire, 1929)
15. Jacobson PD: Medical malpractice and the tort system. JAMA 262:3320–3327, 1989
16. Joint Commission on Accreditation of Health Organizations: Hospital-sponsored ambulatory care services. Oak Brook Terrace, IL, Joint Commission on Accreditation of Health Organizations, 1990, pp 53–63
17. Lehmann TR, Brand RA: Disability in the patient with low back pain. Orthop Clin North Am 13:559–568, 1982
18. Lipkin RJ: Beyond good samaritans and moral monsters: An individualistic justification of the general legal duty to rescue. UCLA Law Review 31:252, 1983
19. Luck JV, Florence DW: A brief history and comparative analysis of disability systems and impairment rating guides. Orthop Clin North Am 19:839–844, 1988
20. May WF: The Physician's Covenant: Images of the Healer in Medical Ethics. Philadelphia, Westminster Press, 1983
21. Smith MA: Importance of satisfactory reporting in the care of patients covered by workers' compensation. South Med J 78:598–601, 1985
22. Thode EW: The unconscious patient: Who should bear the risk of unexplained injuries to a healthy part of his body? Utah Law Review 1:1–12, 1969
23. Thomas V. Corso, 288 A2d 379 (Maryland)
24. US Congress H.R. 3755. Social Security Disability Benefits Reform Act of 1984. 98th Congress, 2nd session. Washington, DC, US Government Printing Office, 1984, Y1.1/8:98–618
25. Ybarra v. Spangler, 154 P2d 687 (California, 1944)
26. Zuger A, Miles SH: Physicians, AIDS, and occupational risk: Historic traditions and ethical obligations. JAMA 258:1924–1928, 1987

Address reprint requests to

Jay Meythaler, JD, MD
Spain Rehabilitation Center
Department of Rehabilitation Medicine
University of Alabama School of Medicine
1717 Sixth Avenue South
Birmingham, AL 35233-7330

MEDICATION AND THE OFFICE MANAGEMENT OF PAIN

F. Peter Buckley, MB, FFARCS, and Charles Chabal, MD

Pain has been defined by the International Association for the Study of Pain as "an unpleasant sensory and emotional experience associated with actual or potential tissue damage, or described in terms of such damage."

The definition continues: "Pain is always subjective. Each individual learns the application of the word through experiences related to injury in early life. It is unquestionably a sensation in a part of the body but is also always unpleasant and therefore an emotional experience. Many people report pain in the absence of tissue damage or any likely pathophysiologic cause, usually this happens for psychologic reasons. There is no way to distinguish their experience from that due to tissue damage, if we take the subjective report. If they regard their experience as pain and if they report it in the same ways as pain caused by tissue damage, it should be accepted as pain. This definition avoids tying pain to the stimulus. Activity induced in the nociceptor and in the nociceptive pathways by a noxious stimulus is not pain, which is always a psychologic state, even though we may well not appreciate that pain most often has a proximate physical cause."

The model in Figure 1 is helpful in conceptualizing aspects of the pain experience. Nociception is the detection of tissue damage by peripheral sensory transducers and centripetal signaling via peripheral nerves. Pain is the recognition of nociceptive signaling by the central nervous system (CNS). Nociceptive signals may originate from periphery (e.g., fracture), from lesions in the spinal cord (e.g., postparaplegia pain) or brain (e.g., thalamic pain syndrome). Suffering is the negative affective response to pain that may also occur in response to, or be heightened by, emotional factors such as fear, anxiety, and depression. Pain behaviors are those things that the sufferer does and says, or does not do or say, and are the only part of this schema that can be observed. These observations, plus data from the history, physical examination, and investigations, enable the clinician to diagnose the sources of the pain and suffering.

From the University of Washington School of Medicine (FPB, CC); Fred Hutchinson Cancer Research Center (FPB); and Veterans Administration Medical Center (CC), Seattle, Washington

PHYSICAL MEDICINE AND REHABILITATION CLINICS OF NORTH AMERICA

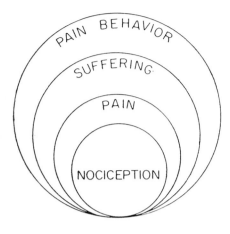

Figure 1. A schematic diagram of the components of pain. (*From* Loeser JD: Concepts of pain. *In* Stanton-Hicks M, Boas R (eds): Chronic Low Back Pain. New York, Raven Press, 1982, p 146; with permission.)

An accurate diagnosis is necessary to select an appropriate pharmacologic therapy. In acute circumstances, in which tissue damage has occurred and nociception is demonstrable, e.g., fracture, an accurate diagnosis is simply made and is certain. The pathophysiology, pharmacology, and nociceptive signaling involved are fairly well understood, and thus, selection of therapies is simple and the therapies are effective. In contrast, our understanding of the processes involved in chronic pain is less comprehensive. Thus, diagnosis is difficult and less certain, selecting therapies is less straightforward, and therapies are often not very effective.

Accurate diagnoses and selection of therapies are important not only to ease the patient's suffering but also to avoid exposing the patient to the idiosyncratic, and drug- and dose-related, side effects of pharmacotherapy. Therapies should be aimed at specific targets for specific reasons, not selected randomly in the hope, rather than the belief, that the therapeutic target may be hit. Therapies should be pursued in a rational pharmacokinetic and pharmacodynamic fashion for a length of time that will give the therapy a reasonable therapeutic trial. Applying the concept of a therapeutic trial is important in patients with chronic pain, in whom the effect of therapies may be uncertain. As in any trial, the results should be monitored by the patient (kept in diary form) and by the physician (appropriate questions and documentation at follow-up visits).

It is tempting for both physician and patient to think that if dose x of a drug is effective, dose 2x will be more effective. Pursuing such a line of reasoning may expose the patient to dose-related side effects because it ignores the fact that some drugs have a ceiling effect and others a therapeutic window. This is worth emphasizing to patients, who, seeking relief and having access to over-the-counter analgesics, may pursue dose escalation and be at risk for dose-related side effects.

NONOPIOID ANALGESICS

Many drugs, both over-the-counter and prescription, are available. They may be grouped into nonsteroidal anti-inflammatory drugs (NSAIDs) and phenacetin derivatives, acetaminophen being the only clinically used drug in the latter category. Information about these agents is given in Table 1.

Table 1. CLASSIFICATION, PHARMACOKINETICS, AND PHARMACOLOGY OF NONOPIOID ANALGESICS

Class and Generic Name	Pharmacologic Properties				Therapeutic Effects*		
	Dosage (mg Orally)	Peak Effect (h)	Duration (h)	Half-life (h)	Analgesic	Anti-inflammatory	Antipyretic
Salicylates							
Aspirin	325–1000 q4–6h	2	4–6	0.25	+++	+++	+++
Choline salicylate	870–1740 q3–4h	0.5–1	>12	(2–30 for salicylate metabolites)	+++	+++	+++
Para-aminophenols							
Acetaminophen	325–1000 q4–6h	0.5–1	4–6	1–4	+++	0	+++
Indoleacetic acid derivatives							
Indomethacin	25–75 q6h	2	6–8	2–3	+++	+++	+++
Sulindac	150–200 q12h	1–2	12	7–18	+++	+++	+++
Pyrazole derivatives							
Phenylbutazone	100–200 q6h	2	6–8	50–100 days	++	++++	++
Oxyphenbutazone	100–200 q6h	2			++	+++	++
Fenmates							
Mefenamic acid	500 q6–8h	2		3–4	++	++	+
Pyrroleacetic acid derivatives							
Tolmetin	200–400 q6–8h	0.5–1		1–3	++	+++	++
Propionic acid derivatives							
Ibuprofen	200–800 q8–12h	1–2	4–6	2	+++	+++	++
Naproxen	250–500 q8–12h	2	8–12	12–15	+++	+++	++
Ketoprofen	50–100 q6–8h	1–2	6	1–35	++	+++	+
Suprofen	200 q4–6h	0.5–1	4	2	+++	++	+
Benzothiazine derivatives							
Piroxicam	20 q12–24h	2–4	24+	45	+++	+++	+

* 0 = no effect; + = minimal effect; ++ = moderate effect; +++ = strong effect; ++++ = maximal effect.

Adapted from Benedetti C, Butler SH: Systemic analgesics. *In* Bonica JJ (ed): The Management of Pain, ed 2. Philadelphia, Lea & Febiger, 1990, pp 1640–1675; with permission.

The pharmacologic effect of NSAIDs is to reduce prostaglandin formation by inhibiting the enzyme cyclooxygenase, part of the arachidonic acid cascade (Fig. 2). Prostaglandins are among the agents released by tissue injury; some stimulate nociceptors or sensitize (or both) nociceptors to the effects of other algogenic agents (bradykinin, histamine, 5-hydroxytryptamine [5-HT]) released by tissue injury. On the basis of cross-perfusion experiments[34] and the analgesia produced by direct injection into inflamed tissue,[16] the major effect of NSAIDs is believed to be peripheral, consistent with the observed efficacy of NSAIDs in pain caused by peripheral inflammation.

Prostaglandins also play some role in the CNS transmission of pain. In animals, noxious stimuli cause their release from the spinal cord[51] and their direct application onto the spinal cord lowers nociceptive thresholds.[68] The direct application of NSAIDs onto the spinal cord reduces peripherally induced nociception in animals and perhaps in humans.[15] In humans, there is evidence that systemic NSAIDs provide analgesia at a supraspinal level.[67] If NSAIDs do have a central effect, they may have a role in treating pain from sources other than peripheral nociception, but in what circumstances and which agents are unclear.

Ketorolac (Toradol)[9]

Ketorolac is a recently introduced parenteral NSAID; an oral form may be available soon. In a postoperative pain model, a 30- to 60-mg dose produces analgesia equivalent to that of 8 to 10 mg IM morphine. The drug has weak anti-inflammatory effects and a spectrum of side effects similar to that of other NSAIDs, and it is unclear whether its predominant effects are peripheral or central. It has been used only in short-term trials.

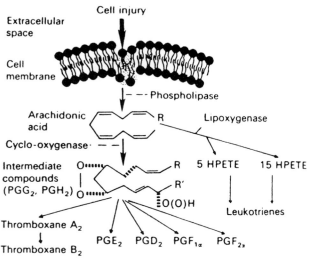

Figure 2. A simplified schema of the genesis of some algogenic agents formed in the arachidonic acid cascade following tissue injury. NSAIDs achieve their peripheral analgesic activity by inhibiting the enzyme cyclooxygenase, which catalyses the formation of prostaglandin precursors from arachidonic acid. (*From* Bonica JJ (ed): The Management of Pain, ed 2. Philadelphia, Lea and Febiger, 1990, p 96; with permission.)

Acetaminophen

Although acetaminophen produces analgesia similar to that of NSAIDs, unlike NSAIDs it has minor anti-inflammatory effects. Acetaminophen is as potent as aspirin in inhibiting prostaglandin synthetase in the CNS but has little effect on prostaglandin metabolism peripherally.[17] In animals, acetaminophen blocks transmission within spinal noradrenergic synapses,[55] depresses nociception transmission at the thalamic level,[11] and interferes with the role of other spinal nociceptive mediators.[27] In humans, acetaminophen produces analgesia via a CNS route, but the actual site of action is unclear.[45]

Side Effects of Nonopioid Analgesics

Nonopioids have a variety of side effects, which are extensively reviewed elsewhere.[31] Briefly, the effects are gastrointestinal intolerance and bleeding (NSAIDs), potential renal toxicity with long-term use of large doses (NSAIDs), and impairment of platelet function (NSAIDs, especially aspirin).

Use of Nonopioid Analgesics

Nonopioid analgesics have a ceiling effect, i.e., increasing doses and blood levels improves analgesia to a certain point, but beyond that point no further benefits occur. Thus, once the recommended dose has been reached and maintained for a certain period of time, increasing the dose does not improve analgesia and increases the occurrence of side effects.

Other than the distinction that NSAIDs suppress inflammation and acetaminophen has few anti-inflammatory effects, there are few data on the comparable efficacy of the various agents. The differences between the agents are in durations of action, degree of side effects, and individual patient tolerance, which should be considered when an agent is selected.

Nonopioid analgesics are suitable for sole use in mild-to-moderate nociceptive and inflammatory pain. Alone, they provide inadequate analgesia for moderate-to-severe nociceptive pain but, if used with opioids, may improve the quality of analgesia and demonstrate an opioid-sparing effect, i.e., reduce the dose of opioid necessary to produce a given level of analgesia.

The place of nonopioid analgesics in the management of neuropathic pain is virtually unstudied and hence unclear; however, the emerging data on the CNS effects of these agents imply that they may have a place.

The role of nonopioids in the management of pain of uncertain origin is unclear. Empiric trials of these agents may be worthwhile, but such trials should be carefully monitored (see earlier discussion), and the ceiling effects and the drugs' long-term liabilities should be borne in mind.

TRICYCLIC ANTIDEPRESSANTS[36, 43]

Many patients with chronic (>6 months' duration) nonmalignant pain are depressed. Pain may be a manifestation of a primary depressive disorder, and thus, pain relief may be a result of antidepressant therapy; however, tricyclic antidepressants (TCAs) appear to have analgesic effects independent of their antidepressant effect, providing pain relief in the nondepressed patient or providing pain relief, without affecting mood, in the depressed patient.[39] Moreover, the analgesic effects of many TCAs occur at dose levels and blood levels of drug lower than those that produce antidepressant effects.

The putative mechanism of effect of the TCAs is an alteration of relative or absolute deficiencies of a number of monoamine transmitters (MA) such as serotonin (5-HT) and norepinephrine (NE) in areas of the CNS that govern mood. TCAs are thought to relieve pain by altering the MA levels in the endorphin-mediated descending antinociceptive system, but the enhancement of which MA (5-HT, NE) is most effective is unclear. In animals, 5-HT–active TCAs appear to be the most effective. In humans, 5-HT specificity is not an absolute criterion. The most widely studied drug, amitriptyline, is relatively 5-HT specific, but it undergoes metabolism to secondary amines, which may inhibit reuptake of NE. In humans, NE enhancement appears to be increasingly important. In peripheral neuropathies in humans, drugs that are 5-HT specific, such as fluoxetine,[41] are ineffective when compared with amitriptyline and drugs that have predominantly an NE effect, such as desipramine.[29, 40, 41] In patients with low back pain, however, doxepin and desipramine have similar efficacy.[65]

Agents and Their Administration

The commonly used TCAs and their pharmacologic profile, side effects, and dosage are given in Table 2.

It is desirable to begin TCA therapy with a low dose, e.g., 10 mg amitriptyline, and titrate upward against side effects, which are often the limiting factor. Low initial doses and slow escalation are important in the elderly, who eliminate these agents slowly. A further tactic is to have the patient take the drug at bedtime so that side effects are less problematic or are useful, e.g., in the case of sedation. All TCAs have long elimination half-lives, and efficacy is not a casualty of once-a-day dosage.

The maintenance dose of TCA is a matter of some contention. The dose levels that produce analgesia are generally lower than those that produce antidepressant effects. For dosage guidelines, see Table 2. The analgesic effects of TCAs are often not seen for 10 to 20 days; thus, it is necessary to continue therapy for several weeks before the therapy can be deemed effective or ineffective.

Conditions in Which TCAs Provide Analgesia

Although the literature is replete with reports of the effects of TCAs in patients with pain, many are questionable because of methodologic deficiencies. The studies quoted in this section are highly selected, placebo-controlled studies in pain states that the physician is likely to encounter in an outpatient practice.

Low Back Pain

Table 3 gives the results of the available trials of TCAs for low back pain. Of the drugs used, none was more effective than placebo, despite use at therapeutic dosages for substantial lengths of time. Possibly, the heterogeneity of the causes of low back pain and the often long duration of pain—in the case of one study,[44] more than 1 year—argue against a demonstration of effectiveness.

Table 2. TRICYCLIC ANTIDEPRESSANTS COMMONLY USED FOR PAIN

Drug	Initial Dosage (mg)	Maintenance Dosage (mg)	Efficacy in Depression*	Adverse and Side Effects*		Biogenic Amine Effect*		Anticholinergic Effect*
				Orthostatic Hypotension	Sedation	5-HT	NE	
Tricyclics								
Amitriptyline	10–300	10–150	++++	++	+++	++++	++	++++
Clomipramine	20–200	20–150	++++	++	++	++++	++	+++
Desipramine	75–300	75–100	++++	++	–	++	++++	+
Doxepin	30–300	30–200	++++	++	++++	++	+	+++
Imipramine	20–300	20–150	++++	+++	+	+++	+++	++
Nortriptyline	50–150	50–150	++++	+	+	++	+++	++
Trimipramine	50–225	75–150	++++	++	+++	+	+	++
Second-generation drugs								
Maprotiline	75–300	75–125	++++	+	++	++	++	+
Trazodone	50–600	100–300	+++	++	+++	++	+	–
Serotonin uptake inhibitors								
Fluoxetine	20–40	20	++++	–	–	++++	–	–

* Value of effects: ++++ = marked; +++ = moderate; ++ = mild; + = minimal; – = absent. Only values in a column should be compared.
5-HT = serotonin; NE = norepinephrine.
Adapted from Monks R: Psychotropic drugs. *In* Bonica JJ (ed): The Management of Pain, ed 2. Philadelphia, Lea & Febiger, 1990, pp 1676–1689; with permission.

Table 3. TRICYCLIC ANTIDEPRESSANTS USED IN PATIENTS WITH LOW BACK PAIN

Reference	Study Design	Type of Rheumatic Pain	Number of Patients	Concomitant Depression	Drug, Dosage (mg/d)	Study Duration (wk)	Results	Other Comments
Jenkins et al, 1976	p	Low back pain	59	15 subjects with high depression scores on BDI	IMI, 75	4	IMI = PL	
Alcoff et al, 1982	p	Low back pain	50	7 patients	IMI, 150	8	IMI > PL on several measures; on pain severity IMI = PL ($P < 0.058$)	No linear relationship between plasma concentrations of IMI and DMI and therapeutic effects
Hameroff et al, 1982	p	Low back pain, cervical pain	30	All patients	DOX, mean of 1.85 mg/kg at week 2, 2.5 mg/kg at week 6	6	DOX = PL on pain severity scores	DOX > PL on depression scores
Pheasant et al, 1983	co	Low back pain	16	All patients with some depression	AMI, 50–150	6	AMI = PL on pain measures	AMI group used significantly less analgesic than PL group

IMI = imipramine; PL = placebo; DOX = doxepin; AMI = amitriptyline; p = parallel; co = crossover; BDI = Beck Depression Inventory.
Adapted from Magni G: The use of antidepressants in the treatment of chronic pain. Drugs 42:730–748, 1991; with permission.

Patients with a short duration of pain are more likely to respond to either doxepin or desipramine than are patients with a long duration of pain.[65]

Osteoarthritis and Rheumatoid Arthritis

Many studies of TCAs in osteoarthritis and rheumatoid arthritis (Table 4) are not very "clean," grouping patients with pain of various causes and, with the exception of one study,[12] against the background of other analgesic therapies. The overall trend is for some modest improvement with TCAs. The study by Caruso and Pietro Grande[12] is particularly interesting: it included high numbers of patients with osteoarthritis in whom ademetionine was similar in efficacy to naproxen and better tolerated with respect to side effects; however, the plateau of efficacy with naproxen was reached in about 15 days, whereas the TCA required approximately 30 days. The results with rheumatoid arthritis were modest at best, even when these agents were combined with other standard therapies.

Fibrositis and Fibromyalgia

All the TCAs used for fibrositis and fibromyalgia produced some benefits (Table 5). The only drug that appeared to be ineffective was maprotiline. Low doses were used in all studies, the onset of benefit occurred after 2 to 3 weeks, and there was agreement among investigators that improvement in pain was closely tied to improvement in mood. At issue on this latter point is whether this improvement was a direct effect of the TCA or an indirect effect of TCAs' improving sleep patterns, which are known to be disturbed in fibrositis and fibromyalgia.

Peripheral Neuropathic Pain

Studies on TCAs in peripheral neuropathic pain (Table 6) concerned either postherpetic neuralgia or diabetic neuropathy. It is probably reasonable to extrapolate the data from these studies to compression or entrapment neuropathies, which are resistant to most therapies.

When compared with placebo, all the TCAs used appear to produce benefits, despite low doses used by some[31, 39, 40] and high doses by others.[29, 53] In all studies, the benefits began after about 2 weeks. There is some suggestion that those patients whose pain responded to the TCA had higher plasma levels of drug, but a frank correlation between blood level of drug and analgesic efficacy has not been established. Amitriptyline is probably the drug of choice, but desipramine is emerging as a satisfactory alternative with similar efficacy and possible fewer side effects.[40, 41]

Central Pain

Only two controlled studies on TCA use for central pain are available. In 18 patients with dysesthetic pain due to a traumatic myelopathy, a 6-week trial of trazodone, 150 mg per day, did not provide any better relief than did placebo.[14] In the second study,[33] 15 patients with poststroke pain were treated with either amitriptyline, 75 mg; carbamazepine, 800 mg per day; or placebo. Carbamazepine and placebo had similar efficacy, and amitriptyline was somewhat superior to placebo. The doses of drug were low, and there was a suggestion that benefit might correlate with higher blood levels of drug; thus, trials with larger doses are in order.

Table 4. TRICYCLIC ANTIDEPRESSANTS USED IN PATIENTS WITH ARTHRITIC CONDITIONS

Reference	Study Design	Type of Rheumatic Pain	Number of Patients	Concomitant Depression	Drug, Dosage (mg/d)	Study Duration (wk)	Results	Other Comments
Thorpe & Marchant-Williams, 1974	p	Arthritis, rheumatoid arthritis	31	Not known	DIB, 240	12	DIB group significantly improved; PL did not improve. No clear statistical comparison of DIB vs. PL	Concomitant analgesic treatment allowed
Gringas, 1976	co	Osteoarthritis, rheumatoid arthritis, ankylosing spondylitis	65	Patients with psychiatric diagnosis excluded	IMI, 50–75	4	IMI > PL	IMI added to standard analgesic antirheumatic therapy
Ganvir et al, 1980	p	Arthritis, rheumatoid arthritis, and other rheumatic conditions	74	Not known	CLO, 25	8	CLO = PL	Concomitant analgesic treatment allowed
Grace et al, 1985	p	Rheumatoid arthritis	36	Not known	AMI, 75	12	AMI = PL	AMI adjunct therapy to other treatments
Caruso & Pietro Grande, 1987	p	Arthritis	734	Not known	SAMe, 1200 NAPROX, 750	4	SAMe > PL; NAPROX > PL	No concomitant treatment allowed
Sarzi Puttini et al, 1988	p	Rheumatoid arthritis	60	30 patients depressed	DOT, 75	4	DOT > PL daytime pain; DOT = PL for nighttime and spontaneous pain	DOT adjunct to IBU 600 mg/d in all subjects
Frank et al, 1988	co	Rheumatoid arthritis	47	Present in some patients, but exact percentage not reported	AMI, 1.5 mg/kg DMI, 1.5 mg/kg TRAZ, 3 mg/kg	6	AMI > PL; DMI, TRAZ = PL; DMI, TRAZ, and PL significantly improved pain symptoms compared with baseline	Investigational treatment adjunct to standard rheumatoid arthritis treatment regimen

IMI = imipramine; PL = placebo; CLO = clomipramine; DIB = dibenzipine; AMI = amitriptyline; DOT = dothiepin; SAMe = S-adenosyl-L-methionine; NAPROX = naproxen; DMI = desipramine; TRAZ = trazodone; IBU = ibuprofen; p = parallel; co = crossover.
Adapted from Magni G: The use of antidepressants in the treatment of chronic pain. Drugs 42:730–748, 1991; with permission.

Table 5. TRICYCLIC ANTIDEPRESSANTS USED IN PATIENTS WITH FIBROSITIS AND FIBROMYALGIA

Reference	Study Design	Type of Rheumatic Pain	Number of Patients	Concomitant Depression	Drug, Dosage (mg/d)	Study Duration (wk)	Results	Other Comments
Bibolotti et al, 1986	co	Fibrositis	37	Some depressive symptoms present in all patients	MAP, 75; CLO, 75	3	CLO significantly improved number of trigger points from baseline, MAP did not; PL significantly worsened number of trigger points from baseline. No clear comparison between active drugs and PL	High percentage of drop-outs in the CLO group
Carette et al, 1986	p	Primary fibrositis	70	Not known	AMI 50	9	AMI > PL for patient and physician global assessment. No statistical difference between AMI and PL for pain scores	
Goldenberg et al, 1986	p	Primary fibrositis	62	Not known	NAPROX, 1000; NAPROX + AMI, 1000 + 25; AMI, 25	6	AMI > PL; NAPROX = PL	
Caruso et al, 1987	p	Primary fibrositis	60	Not known	DOT, 75	8	DOT > PL	
Tavoni et al, 1987	co	Primary fibrositis	25	11 of 17 patients who completed the trial had some depression	SAMe, 200 IM	3	SAMe significantly decreased number of tender points, PL did not. No clear comparison between the 2 groups	Improvement of pain linked to improvement in depression

MAP = maprotiline; CLO = clomipramine; DOT = dothiepin; AMI = amitriptyline; NAPROX = naproxen; SAMe = S-adenosyl-L-methionine; p = parallel; co = crossover.

Adapted from Magni G: The use of antidepressants in the treatment of chronic pain. Drugs 42:730–748, 1991; with permission.

Table 6. SOME PLACEBO-CONTROLLED STUDIES OF ANTIDEPRESSANTS IN THE TREATMENT OF PATIENTS WITH PERIPHERAL NEUROPATHIC PAIN

Reference	Study Design	Type of Pain	Number of Patients	Concomitant Depression	Drug, Dosage (mg/d)	Study Duration (wk)	Results	Other Comments
Watson et al, 1982	co	Postherpetic neuralgia	24	9 patients	AMI, 25–137.5; median 75 mg for 16 responders, 50 mg for 8 nonresponders	3	AMI > PL	Effects seem to persist in the long term (1 yr), analgesic effect independent of antidepressant action
Kvinesdal et al, 1984	co	Diabetic neuropathy	15	Not known	IMI, 100	5	IMI > PL	Some relation between plasma concentrations of the drug and response
Max et al, 1987	co	Diabetic neuropathy	37	14 of the 29 patients who completed the study	AMI, 25–150: mean 90	6	AMI ≥ PL	Responders had higher plasma concentrations for AMI and NORT
Sindrup et al, 1989	co	Diabetic neuropathy	13	Not known	IMI, 125–225; mean 177	3	IMI > PL	Effect not mediated by change in mood
Kishore-Kumar et al, 1990	co	Postherpetic neuralgia	26	4 patients	DMI, mean dosage 168 at week 5, 167 at week 6	6	DMI > PL	
Max et al, 1991	co	Diabetic neuropathy	20	7/20 depressed	DMI, mean 201 mg	12	DMI > PL	Pain relief greater in depressed patients
Max et al, 1992	co	Diabetic neuropathy	57	15/57	AMI, mean 105; DMI, mean 111; FLUOX, mean 40	8	AMI = DMI > FLUOX = PL	AMI + DMI effective in both depressed and nondepressed, no correlation between benefits and serum drug levels

AMI = amitriptyline; DMI = desipramine; IMI = imipramine; FLUOX = fluoxetine; PL = placebo; co = crossover.
Adapted from Magni G: The use of antidepressants in the treatment of chronic pain. Drugs 42:730–748; 1991; with permission.

OPIOIDS

Drugs that produce analgesia through direct effects on CNS receptors, of which morphine is the prototype, are colloquially referred to as narcotic analgesics. It is helpful to refer to these drugs as *opioids* rather than *narcotics*, which semantically associates them with opium, the source of the prototype drug, morphine. This terminology is advised for a number of reasons. Narcotic is a legislative, administrative, or legal word applied to a number of psychoactive drugs with abuse potential, including not only therapeutically useful agents such as opioids but also agents (such as cocaine) with minimal therapeutic usefulness. In the current social and legislative atmosphere ("just say no", the "war on drugs") the word *narcotic* carries the stigma of association with the dire personal, social, and health consequences of the use of such psychoactive drugs by the drug-addict population. Therefore, because of their association with addiction, many of the public, and some health care professionals, are wary of the use of opioids, even when their use is absolutely appropriate, rational, medically and socially sanctioned, and safe, e.g., for postoperative analgesia. The avoidance of such opioids by patients or health care professionals in circumstances in which they should be appropriately used is to do a grave disservice to those suffering from treatable pain. Although it is the duty of the medical profession to recognize the usefulness and low risks of opioids and to use them appropriately, it is unlikely that public concern about the risks of opioids, however erroneous, will abate in the near future.

Opioids produce analgesia by acting at a number of different levels of the CNS:

1. Opioids inhibit the transmission of nociceptive input from the periphery in the dorsal horn of the spinal cord. This probably only occurs with high cerebrospinal fluid (CSF) concentrations of opioid, e.g., after intraspinal injection, and probably plays a minor role in the analgesia produced by systemic drug administration.
2. Opioids activate descending inhibitory systems in the basal ganglia that modulate peripheral nociceptive input at the spinal cord level. This activation occurs at low CSF concentrations of drug and is the most likely mechanism of analgesia produced by systemic opioids.
3. Opioids function in the limbic system by altering the emotional response to pain, thereby making it more bearable.

The receptors to which opioids bind, the agents that prototypically activate them, and the effects of receptor activation are given in Table 7. The receptor binding of opiates in common clinical use is given in Table 8.

Opioids that bind to receptors and produce effects are termed *agonists;* morphine is the classic μ agonist. Some opioids, e.g., naloxone, bind to receptors and yet produce no effect; these drugs are termed *antagonists.* Antagonists block the effects of a subsequently administered agonist and partially reverse the effect of a previously administered agonist, potentially precipitating a withdrawal syndrome in a patient who is physically dependent on opioid agonists.

Other opioids are agonists at one receptor and antagonists at another, e.g., nalbuphine, a μ antagonist and a κ agonist that can antagonize the μ effects of morphine yet still retains some of the κ effects of nalbuphine. These agents are termed agonist/antagonists.

Opioids exert a dose-dependent analgesic effect and can control pain as great as that caused by surgical procedures. The major limiting factor in the use of

Table 7. OPIATE RECEPTOR EFFECTS

μ_1	μ_2	κ	σ	δ
Morphine β-Endorphin		Bremazocine Dynorphin	N-allylcyclazocine	Morphine Leu-enkephalin
Analgesia	No analgesia	Analgesia	No analgesia	No analgesia
Apnea (?)	Apnea	Apnea ±	Tachypnea	Apnea + +
Indifference	Sedation	Sedation	Delirium	?
Miosis		Miosis	Mydriasis	
Nausea and vomiting				Nausea and vomiting
Constipation				
Urine retention		Diuresis		
Pruritus		No change	No change	Pruritus
Change in temperature				
δ Cross-tolerance		No cross-tolerance		μ Cross-tolerance

Adapted from Benedetti C: Acute pain: A review of its effects and therapy with systemic opioids. *In* Benedetti C, Chapman CR, Giron G (eds): Opioid Analgesia: Recent Advances in Systemic Administration. (Advances in Pain Research and Therapy, vol 14.) New York, Raven Press, 1990, pp 367–424; with permission.

opioids is that unwanted effects (sedation, respiratory depression) occur with rising blood levels of the drug. The analgesic dose-response curve of opioids is not a straight line; they have a threshold of efficacy and a narrow "therapeutic window" (Fig. 3).

The blood level of drug at which pain ceases to be felt has been termed the *minimum effective analgesic concentration* (MEAC).[3] For an individual patient with a

Table 8. OPIATE RECEPTOR INTERACTIONS

Drug	Receptor			
	μ	κ	σ	δ
Morphine	+ + +	+		+ +
Fentanyl	+ + + +			+
Meperidine	+ +			+ +
Hydromorphone	+ + +			+ +
Methadone	+ + +			+ +
Naloxone	− − −	−	−	−
Naloxazone	− − − −			
Nalbuphine	− − −	+ + +	+	
Pentazocine	−	+ + +	+ +	?
Nalorphine		+ +	+ + +	+ +
Butorphanol		+ +	+ +	

+ = agonist effect; − = antagonist effect.
Adapted from Benedetti C: Acute pain: A review of its effects and therapy with systemic opioids. *In* Benedetti C, Chapman CR, Giron G (eds): Opioid Analgesia: Recent Advances in Systemic Administration. (Advances in Pain Research and Therapy, vol 14.) New York, Raven Press, 1990, pp 367–424; with permission.)

PLASMA MEPERIDINE (Micrograms/ml)

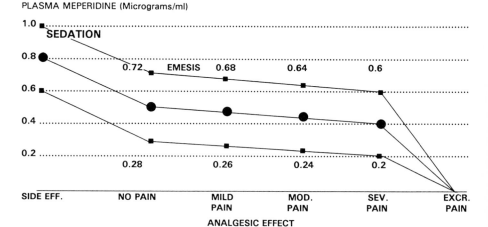

Figure 3. Mean plasma levels of meperidine plus 1 standard deviation above and below the mean, plotted against pain relief. The relation between plasma concentration and pain relief is not linear. Until a certain plasma level is reached, in this case a mean of 0.4 μg/mL, little pain relief is achieved. Above this plasma level, analgesia improves linearly to a plasma level of about 0.5 μg/mL, a level at which there is no pain. Around and above this plasma level, side effects—emesis and sedation—become more pronounced. Thus, in this case, the "therapeutic window" for meperidine is narrow and consists of mean plasma levels from 0.4 to 0.5 μg/mL. Note the wide standard deviations, which reflect large individual variations in drug effect (see text). (*Modified from* Benedetti C: Acute pain: A review of its effects and therapy with systemic opioids. *In* Benedetti C, Chapman CR, Giron G (eds): Advances in Pain Research and Therapy, vol 14. New York, Raven Press, 1990, pp 367–424; with permission.)

given pain, the MEAC is very consistent[22]; however, individual patients with similar pains have MEACs that vary over a five to six fold range. The mean MEAC of morphine is 16 ng/mL, SD 9, range 6 to 33, and the mean MEAC for meperidine is 455 ng/mL, SD 174, range 94 to 754.[4] This information, allied with the individually variable drug half-lives and speeds of elimination, means that among patients a wide range of doses of opioids is necessary to maintain blood levels close to MEAC and thus effective analgesia. The corollary of this is that the doses of opioids used to provide analgesia must be individualized, based on the effects of the drug, which in practice means patient report.

Opioids have a wide variety of side effects. Gastrointestinal effects include slowing of gastric emptying and intestinal transit. Genitourinary effects are increased tone and contractility of the ureter and increased detrusor tone leading to urinary retention. CNS effects include sedation, euphoria or dysphoria, respiratory depression, nausea, and vomiting.

Tolerance is a normal response to opioid therapy and is the progressively decreasing effect (analgesia or other effects) to a given dose of drug. Tolerance is a drug-related effect only and bears little relation to addiction, and its occurrence says nothing about the individual patient's predilection to becoming psychologically dependent on the drug. The clinical scenario in which tolerance is seen is that a patient who has been achieving good analgesia with a given dose progressively fails to do so, with no evidence of changing nociception. Tolerance may be overcome by increasing the dose of drug or partially overcome by switching to another drug.

Physical dependence is also a normal response to opioid therapy and is characterized by the occurrence of an abstinence syndrome (yawning, lacrimation, sneezing, agitation, tremors, fever, tachycardia, and other signs of sympathetic arousal) if the opioid is abruptly withdrawn. Like tolerance, dependence is a drug, not a patient, characteristic and is an entity separate from addiction. Addicts may be opioid dependent, but few patients who are opioid dependent are addicts (see later discussion). Withdrawal syndromes can be avoided by slow reduction of opioid dose (10%–20% per day) or by using α_2-adrenergic agonists such as clonidine. An opioid withdrawal syndrome is very unpleasant but, unlike alcohol or sedative withdrawal, is very rarely life threatening.

Psychological dependence (addiction) is characterized by an abnormal pattern of drug use; of drug craving for effects other than pain relief; by an overwhelming involvement with procuring and consuming the drug, even when such activity is contrary to the individual's best interests; and with a tendency to relapse into drug use after withdrawal. The overwhelming body of opinion is that addiction is the conjunction of genetic, psychological, social, and cultural factors affecting an individual, in addition to use of the drug. In short, unlike tolerance and physical dependence, psychological dependence is patient issue, not a drug issue. Patients with no previous history of substance abuse who received opioids therapeutically have a low incidence of iatrogenic addiction, approximately 1 in 2000 to 4000.[50] Therefore, in patients with no history of substance abuse, fear of producing psychological dependence should not be a major factor in restricting the use of opioids in appropriate circumstances.

Commonly Used Opioids

A list of commonly used opioids and their approximate equianalgesic doses, half-lives, and dosage intervals is given in Table 9. The choice of agent depends on the severity of pain, the drugs with which the physician is familiar, and desired dosing intervals. The choice of agent should be limited to opioid agonists, because the agonist/antagonist drugs have few real advantages.

The pharmacokinetic and pharmacodynamic properties of opioids dictate their rational use. The target is to reach the patient's MEAC, a blood level of drug that provides analgesia without side effects, and then to maintain the blood level at or about that level for the desired length of time. In practice this means giving initial loading doses and then repeat doses at regular intervals, consistent with the drug's duration of effect; however, given the wide range of individual variability of dose requirements, therapy should be monitored and adjusted constantly to achieve the desired effect.

Opioid Use in Clinical Practice

There is general agreement that in pain scenarios in which nociception is pronounced, the use of opioids is absolutely appropriate; they provide effective analgesia, acceptable incidence and severity of side effects, and a low incidence of psychological dependence. These scenarios are (1) pain due to acute visceral or somatic damage—classical instances are postoperative and posttrauma pain; and (2) pain due to chronic visceral or somatic damage caused by neoplasms.

Table 9. PHARMACOKINETIC AND PHARMACODYNAMIC DATA OF OPIOID ANALGESICS USED FOR MODERATE-TO-SEVERE PAIN

Class, Generic Name, Proprietary Name	Route	Equianalgesic Dose (mg)	Peak (h)	Duration (h)	Half-life (h)	Comments	Precautions
Agonists—naturally occurring opium derivatives							
Morphine	IM	10–15	0.5–1	3–5	2–3.5	Standard of comparison for opioid-type analgesics	Impaired ventilation, increased intracranial pressure
	PO	30–60	1.5–2	4			
Codeine	IM	120	0.5–1	4–6	3	Less potent than morphine; excellent oral potency	Like morphine
	PO	200		3–4			
Hydromorphone (Dilaudid)	IM	1–2	0.5–1	3–4	2–3	Like heroin	Like morphine
	PO	2–4	1.5–2	4–6			
Oxycodone	PO	30	1	4–6	NA		Like morphine
Methadone (Dolophine)	IM	8–10	0.5–1	4–8	15–30		
	PO	10	1.5–2	4–12			
Propoxyphene HCl (Darvon)	PO	32–65		4–6	3.5	"Weak" opioid, often used in combination with nonopioid analgesics	
Meperidine (Demerol)	IM	75–100	0.5–1	2–3		Shorter acting and about 10% as potent as morphine; has mild atropinelike antispasmodic effects	
	PO	200–300	1–2	2–3			
Fentanyl	IV	50–100		0.75–1		Short-acting potent opioid; mostly used in anesthesia	
Agonist-antagonists							
Buprenorphine (Temgesic)	IM	0.3–0.6	0.5–1	6–8	NA	Partial agonist of the morphine type; less abuse liability than morphine	
	SL	0.4–0.8	2–3	6–8			
Butorphanol (Stadol)	IM	2	0.5–1	4	2.5–3.5	Like nalbuphine	
Pentazocine (Talwin)	IM	40–60	0.5–1	3–4	2–3	Mixed agonist-antagonist; less abuse liability than morphine	
	PO	50–200	1.5–2	3–4			
Nalbuphine (Nubain)	IM	10–20	0.5–1	4–6	5	μ-antagonist and κ-agonist; possibly mild σ-agonist	

Equianalgesic doses to morphine, 10–15 mg IM.
IM = intramuscular; PO = oral; IV = intravenous; SL = sublingual.
Adapted from Benedetti C, Butler SH: Systemic analgesics. *In* Bonica JJ (ed): The Management of Pain, ed 2. Philadelphia, Lea & Febiger, 1990, pp 1640–1675; with permission.

In other clinical pain scenarios, opioids are of little assistance and are relatively contraindicated or controversial: (1) pain due to peripheral neurologic injury such as peripheral neuropathies, causalgias, reflex sympathetic dystrophies[2, 42]; (2) pain due to central neurologic injuries to the spinal cord or brain; and (3) chronic pain of uncertain origin. The most common scenario can be loosely described as chronic musculoskeletal pain in which nociceptive pathology cannot be demonstrated, at least by currently available clinical and technologic means.

In these three groups of patients, there is considerable controversy over whether opioids provide long-term analgesia without untoward sequelae and whether chronic opioid therapy should be used. This controversy deserves further attention.

Against the Chronic Use of Opioids[18, 62]

One side of this controversy, supported by those who work mainly in the behavioral-based management of patients with chronic nonmalignant pain of uncertain origin, holds that opioids are inappropriate in the management of chronic nonmalignant pain. There are several arguments cited to support this position.

1. The belief that the complaint of chronic pain is likely not indicative of nociception but more a product of a variety of internal and environmental contingencies that have been learned and, in this particular context, may be reinforced by the repetitive use of biomedical maneuvers, e.g., opioid prescription and consumption.[18]
2. The belief that the best measures of outcome of therapies are not what the patient says ("I hurt" or "I don't hurt") but more how the patient functions (what he or she does or does not do), which are the data points used as the outcome variables in studies of outcome in behavioral type programs. This group freely admits that patients treated in behaviorally based programs often function well yet complain of pain.
3. Pharmacologically, opioids are effective in treating pain due to nociception. If nociception is not present or cannot be demonstrated to be present, opioids are not an appropriate choice of therapy, and their use may expose patients to the undesirable effects of opioid therapy.
4. Clinical experience to date with patients with chronic nonmalignant pain, who are taking opioids. Approximately 60% of patients referred to pain clinics[54] or admitted to inpatient programs[8, 38, 63] are consuming opioids yet are still in pain and disabled.
5. The retrospective clinical reports of the results of pain-management programs imply that opioids are part of the problem rather than part of the solution and that many patients' complaints improve when safely and appropriately weaned from opioids alone.[7, 37, 38] The reason for the improvement is that opioids are believed to produce a variety of undesirable CNS and psychological states (impaired cognitive function, depression, poor motivation),[37] acting as a reinforcer of sick behaviors[18] and maintaining patients' chronic pain complaints, and what the patients may be experiencing is a minor withdrawal syndrome, which is being labeled by the patient as pain.[7, 25]
6. As many physicians treating patients with this sort of pain are aware, the issue of opioids versus no opioids often becomes the focal issue of patient–physician interactions, thus detracting attention and effort from

other worthwhile endeavors such as progress in therapy or return to work.

7. In the only randomized blinded trial of an opioid (codeine, 60 mg three times daily) against a nonopioid (acetaminophen, 1.0 g three times daily) in a population with chronic nonmalignant pain (hip osteoarthritis), opioids did not produce superior analgesia and had a high incidence of side effects, leading to a high drop-out rate in those treated with opioids.[30]

8. Unspoken is the issue that the use of opioids in these circumstances may be maintaining a substance-use habit rather than dealing with pain treatment.

For the Use of Chronic Opioid Therapy for Chronic Pain[46]

The other side of the controversy, which is supported by those working in the field of cancer-pain management, who are concerned with the ready availability of opioids for cancer therapy, presents a biomedical and moral view of the issue. This view is that pain is a symptom caused by an underlying disease (diagnosed or, in the case in point, often not diagnosable) and thus should be treated in accordance with classic biomedical treatments, i.e., opioids. Moreover, they advance the moral argument that it is the responsibility of the physician to alleviate suffering, and their contention is that this can be achieved, without undue problems, with chronic opioid therapy. The arguments cited in support of this position include the following:

1. It is accepted that opioids are appropriate and safe therapies for cancer pain and postoperative pain, so why not for chronic nonmalignant pain?

2. Virtually all physicians who treat patients with this sort of pain have a coterie of patients whom they maintain on therapy with opioids, at various dosages without apparent ill effects for long periods of time.

3. There have been reports of the successful use of opioids in patients with chronic nonmalignant pain published by the protagonists of this position.[49, 56, 58–60, 69]

These studies are retrospective reports of relatively small groups of patients with pain of various origins who have failed to previously benefit from other therapies. The studies are without clear patient-selection criteria; without clear criteria for benefit of the therapy, other than patient report of relief of pain; and concern patients who were followed up for varying periods of time. Certain useful information has emerged from these studies. Tolerance and toxicity were minor issues. The studies claimed that approximately 60% of patients achieved pain relief benefits, but there were few gains in the social or employment spheres. In most reports there was a low (3%–5%) incidence of so-called problem patients, often those with a previous substance-use history.

The protagonists of this line of reasoning do not dismiss the goals of their antagonists but accommodate to them somewhat, not espousing that chronic opioid therapy is a route for all patients but that a selected group of patients may achieve benefits. Proposed guidelines for selecting patients with chronic nonmalignant pain for chronic opioid therapy have been published and are given in Table 10. Although these guidelines seem reasonable, certain issues emerge if they are followed to the letter:

1. What constitutes reasonable attempts at therapy? Failure to profit from a high-quality pain management program?

Table 10. PROPOSED GUIDELINES IN THE MANAGEMENT OF OPIOID
MAINTENANCE THERAPY FOR NONMALIGNANT PAIN

1. Should be considered only after all other reasonable attempts at analgesia have failed.
2. A history of substance abuse should be viewed as a relative contraindication.
3. A single practitioner should take primary responsibility for treatment.
4. Patients should give informed consent before the start of therapy; points to be covered include recognition of the low risk of psychologic dependence as an outcome, potential for cognitive impairment with the drug alone and in combination with sedative/hypnotics, and understanding by female patients that children born when the mother is on opioid maintenance therapy will likely be physically dependent at birth.
5. After drug selection, doses should be given on an around-the-clock basis; several weeks should be agreed upon as the period of initial dose titration, and although improvement in function should be continually stressed, all should agree to at least partial analgesia as the appropriate goal of therapy.
6. Failure to achieve at least partial analgesia at relatively low initial doses in the nontolerant patient raises questions about the potential treatability of the pain syndrome with opioids.
7. Emphasis should be given to attempts to capitalize on improved analgesia by gains in physical and social function.
8. In addition to the daily dose determined initially, patients should be permitted to escalate dose transiently on days of increased pain; two methods are acceptable: (a) Prescription of an additional 4–6 "rescue doses" to be taken as needed during the month. (b) Instruction that one or two extra doses may be taken on any day, but must be followed by an equal reduction of dose on subsequent days.
9. Most patients should be seen and drugs prescribed at least monthly. Patients should be assessed for the efficacy of treatment, adverse drug effects, and the appearance of either misuse or abuse of the drugs during each visit. The results of the assessment should be clearly documented in the medical record.
10. Exacerbations of pain not effectively treated by transient, small increases in dose are best managed in the hospital, where dose escalation, if appropriate, can be observed closely, and return to baseline doses can be accomplished in a controlled environment.
11. Evidence of drug hoarding, acquisition of drugs from other physicians, uncontrolled dose escalation, or other aberrant behaviors should be followed by tapering and discontinuation of opioid maintenance therapy.

From Portenoy RK: Chronic opioid therapy for nonmalignant pain. Journal of Pain and Symptom Management 5: 558, 1990; with permission. Copyright 1990 by the US Cancer Pain Relief Committee.

2. If failure to profit from extensive attempts at therapy is accepted as a criterion, the numbers of patients eligible would likely be quite small.
3. If a history of substance abuse is viewed as only a relative contraindication, the physician who espouses this treatment philosophy will undoubtedly be able to acquire a wide experience of its advisability from the plentiful supply of such patients who will beat a path to his or her door.
4. If treatment is undertaken by a single practitioner who understands the issues, that physician's time will be taken up largely with such patients. Again, this will render the number of treated patients as being small.

A Middle-Ground View[13]

It is obvious that there is a lack of firm consensus about the effectiveness, safety, and desirability of long-term opioid treatment for chronic nonmalignant pain and that much research needs to be done to define the place, or lack of place, of these agents in this circumstance. While such definition is taking place, what can the clinician offer as a reasonable attempt at therapy in patients with chronic nonmalignant pain in whom opioids may or may not be an issue? An approach, termed by its authors a *biopsychosocial model,* has been proposed. This incorporates elements of the preceding two positions and, like them, remains to be confirmed.

1. New patients are evaluated appropriately to rule out undiscovered biomedical illness.
2. The patient is involved in treatment planning and agrees to participate in a mutually agreed-on pain-management program that emphasizes improved function and decreased suffering but does not promise complete pain relief.
3. Patients are seen at regular intervals as long as the patient and treating physician agree that this is useful.
4. Patients who are not taking opioids when initially seen are rarely prescribed opioids. The place of adjunctive medications and treatments is emphasized.
5. With the patient's consent, the treating physician assumes the responsibility of being the sole prescriber of analgesics and contacts other health care providers caring for the patient to gather information and to alert them to this arrangement.
6. Patients who are taking opioids at the initial visit have their opioid consumption converted to a "pain cocktail" (see later). Patients are informed that this is the only manner in which the physician will prescribe opioids.
7. It is emphasized that the pain cocktail will likely not provide complete pain relief but will be used to ameliorate pain and that the physician will not respond to opioid tolerance by increasing the opioid dose in the pain cocktail.
8. The importance of alternative nonopioid pain management strategies, e.g., relaxation training, exercise, employment, and productive activity, is emphasized, and continued pain cocktail prescription is contingent on participation in these strategies.
9. One of the treatment goals is discontinuation or reduction of opioid intake and perhaps that of other medications. The amount of opioid is tapered over weeks or months, using the pain cocktail in coordination with other treatment modalities.
10. Medication misuse, e.g., excessive consumption and seeking opioids from other sources, is confronted. The physician may respond by increasing the frequency of contact or, at the worst end of the spectrum, requiring the patient to participate in substance-abuse treatment. If these steps are not successful, opioids are tapered at a rate at which a withdrawal syndrome will not occur.
11. Some patients are never completely weaned from opioids but continue taking modest amounts for long periods (are these the patients analogous to those described by Portenoy et al[46]?), with a view to maintaining

quality of life. At the same time, the physician constantly attempts to shift the emphasis of treatment from opioids to other treatment or condition issues.

Medication Weaning

If a physician wishes to reduce or eliminate a patient's opioid consumption, how may this be safely and effectively achieved? Certain factors need to be taken into consideration.

Opioid Pharmacology

The patient may be physically dependent on opioid, i.e., abrupt cessation of opioid intake may precipitate a withdrawal syndrome. Thus, for both humanitarian and treatment-success reasons, any weaning process should minimize the possibility of a withdrawal syndome, and such a syndrome should be treated if it arises.

Patient Factors

The patient may be fearful of a withdrawal syndrome. It can be avoided in the majority of cases by the weaning strategies outlined later. In weaning off opioids, one of the patients' psychic crutches (albeit an ineffectual and perhaps harmful one) is being removed. It is therefore essential that the patient be furnished with alternative measures.

Medications as a Behavioral Factor

In behavioral terms, popping a pill, particularly a pill that is initially likely to produce pleasant psychic effects, is a very effective way to condition a patient to consume pills as a way of coping with a problem.

Practical Realities of Weaning

Initially, the type and magnitude of a patient's opioid consumption must be established. This can be done by perusal of physician or pharmacy records of prescriptions or, perhaps most effectively, by having the patient maintain a diary of type, dose, and frequency of opioid consumption for 1 to 2 weeks. With that information, the patient's mean daily opioid consumption can be ascertained. The presumption is that at this dose level the patient avoids a withdrawal syndrome and therefore this is the logical place to start an opioid wean. When beginning an opioid wean, it is common practice to set the initial daily dose somewhat higher (10%–20%) than that calculated from the diaries.

Weaning from opioids can be achieved in a variety of manners. The most obvious and simple is the pill count method. The patient is prescribed sufficient drug of choice (i.e., that which the patient customarily takes), based on mean daily consumption, to last a given period (from a few days to a week) and is instructed to take them on a time-contingent basis rather than a symptom-contingent basis, consistent with the duration of action of the drug. For example, if the patient takes a mean of 12 oxycodone tablets, 5 mg per day, the initial prescription is for 14 oxycodone tablets a day, 2 tablets taken every 3 to 4 hours. Provided that all has gone well the following week, the wean is commenced and the dose is reduced by 10% to 20%, a reduction that continues until the patient is no longer taking opioids. It is made clear to the patient that it is the duty of the physician to prescribe responsibly and that it is the duty of the patient to consume responsibly. Each prescription must last the appropriate time, and no further prescriptions are forthcoming until the next scheduled refill.

The pill count method has some inherent advantages: The patient can tolerate the drug, and it is simple. There are some disadvantages: The dosages are restricted by pill size; it may be difficult to use a time-contingent strategy with short-acting drugs; and because of the obvious pill count, the patient may become anxious about the reducing number of pills and may become fearful of withdrawal.

An alternative to the pill count method is the pain cocktail strategy.[8, 25] In this strategy, the patient's mean daily intake of opioid is combined into a set volume of a taste-masked liquid vehicle, e.g., cherry syrup, and the volume is split into a number of doses, each dose being prescribed at an interval appropriate to the expected duration of action of the drug. When the opioid content is reduced, the total daily volume stays stable but the opioid content in milligrams is reduced by 10% to 20%.

Just as alcoholic cocktails can contain a variety of ingredients (such as whiskey or gin), so can pain cocktails contain a variety of opioids (short-acting: oxycodone; or long-acting: methadone). The essential premise is that the pain-cocktail dose should be administered at an interval consistent with the duration of action of its opioid drug content.

The original description of the pain cocktail contained methadone as the opioid, selected because of its long action and slow elimination, which are believed to produce a relative lack of "high"; a "smooth" wean; and its ready availability. Use of a methadone pain cocktail requires that the mean daily opioid consumption is converted to methadone, using the opioid equivalences given in Table 11. Thus, for a patient who consumes twelve 5-mg oxycodone tablets (60 mg) per day, the equivalent amount of methadone is 20 mg. This 20 mg is placed in a 40 mL vehicle, and 10 mL is prescribed for every 6 hours. If the physician wishes to use oxycodone as the opioid content, by using the aforementioned example, 60 mg oxycodone would be incorporated in a 60 mL vehicle, and 10 mL would be administered every 4 hours. Whichever opioid is used in the pain cocktail, the frequency of dosage should be consistent with the duration of action of the opioid. When the time comes to reduce, the opioid content of each dose is reduced by 10% to 20% but the same volume of vehicle is administered.

Table 11. ORAL NARCOTIC EQUIANALGESIC DOSES

	mg	Half-life $t_{1/2}$(h)
Methadone	10	22–25
Meperidine	150	3–4
Morphine	30	2–3
Hydromorphone	4	2–4
Oxycodone	15	2–3
Codeine	100	3–4
Dextropropoxyphene HCl	160	6–12
Dextropropoxyphene napsylate	250	6–12

From Sammons EE: Drug use and misuse in chronic pain patients. Clinics in Anaesthesiology 3:176, 1985.

Table 12. ORAL TRANQUILIZER EQUIANALGESIC DOSES

	mg	Half-life $t_{1/2}$(h)
Diazepam	10	20–50
Chlordiazepoxide	20	5–30
Phenobarbital	30	6–8
Oxazepam	30	5–20
Lorazepam	2	10–15
Clorazepate	15	30–100
Prazepam	20	30–100
Alprazolam	1	12–15
Flurazepam	30	47–100
Temazepam	30	9–12
Triazolam	0.5	1.7–3
Alcohol	30*	1.5–2

* Alcohol equianalgesic dose in milliliters rather than milligrams.
From Sammons EE: Drug use and misuse in chronic pain patients. Clinics in Anaesthesiology 3:176, 1985.

Experience with the pain cocktail strategy, predominantly with inpatients,[8] is that it is a safe and effective way of weaning patients from opioids as well as other psychoactive medications. Patients who might be unsuitable for initiating outpatient weaning include those with a previous history of substance use, those consuming relatively large amounts of opioids (>20 mg methadone or its equivalent per day), and those with a history of using intramuscular opioids. In these cases, admission to hospital, initiation of the wean, and continuation as outpatient is probably more appropriate.

The pain cocktail strategy may be used to wean patients from other psychoactive medications, e.g., barbiturates and benzodiazepines. The strategies are very similar to those in weaning from opioids, i.e., the patient's baseline consumption is ascertained; this intake is converted to the classical sedative content of the pain cocktail, phenobarbital (chosen, like methadone, because of its long half-life), from the sedative equivalences in Table 12; and weaning is commenced. Weaning patients from benzodiazepines and barbiturates is somewhat more hazardous than is weaning from opioids. With an opioid wean, the patient may develop a withdrawal syndrome, which, although undoubtedly unpleasant, is not hazardous to health and well being; however, if withdrawal from benzodiazepines and barbiturates proceeds too quickly, the patient may be at risk for convulsions. Hence, this argues against weaning outside a hospital or a specialized treatment facility.

SUMMARY

There is a wide variety of pharmacologic agents available to treat the various pain problems that are encountered in a physical medicine and rehabilitation office practice. The effective and safe prescription and use of these agents requires that their pharmacology, indications and contraindications, side effects, and complications be understood and taken into account. These agents should be used specifically for specific problems, and their use and complications should be closely monitored.

References

1. Alcoff J, Jones E, Rust P, et al: Controlled trial of imipramine for chronic low back pain. J Fam Pract 14:841–846, 1982
2. Arner S, Meyerson BA: Lack of analgesic effect of opioids on neuropathic and idiopathic forms of pain. Pain 33:11–23, 1988
3. Austin KL, Stapleton JV, Mather LE: Relationship of meperidine concentration and analgesic response: A preliminary report. Anesthesiology 53:460–466, 1980
4. Benedetti C: Acute pain: A review of its effects and therapy with systemic opioids. *In* Benedetti C, Chapman CR, Giron G (eds): Opioid Analgesia: Recent Advances in Systemic Administration. (Advances in Pain Research and Therapy, vol 14). New York, Raven Press, 1990, pp 367–424
5. Benedetti C, Butler SH: Systemic analgesics. *In* Bonica JJ (ed): The Management of Pain, ed 2. Philadelphia, Lea & Febiger, 1990, pp 1640–1675
6. Bibolotti E, Borghi C, Pasculli E, et al: The management of fibrositis: A double blind comparison of maprotiline (Ludiomil), chlorimipramine and placebo. Clinical Trials Journal 23:269–280, 1986
7. Black RG: The chronic pain syndrome. Surg Clin North Am 55:999–1011, 1975
8. Buckley FP, Sizemore WE, Charlton JE: Medication management in patients with chronic nonmalignant pain: A review of the use of a drug withdrawal protocol. Pain 26:153–165, 1986
9. Buckley MM-T, Brogden RN: Ketorolac: A review of its pharmacodynamic and pharmacokinetic properties and therapeutic potential. Drugs 39:86–109, 1990
10. Carette S, McCain GA, Bell DA, et al: Evaluation of amitriptyline in primary fibrositis: A double blind, placebo controlled study. Arthritis Rheum 29:655–659, 1986
11. Carlsson KH, Jurna I: Central analgesic effect of paracetamol manifested by depression of nociceptive activity in thalamic neurons of the rat. Neurosci Lett 77:339–343, 1987
12. Caruso I, Pietro Grande V: Italian double-blind multicenter study comparing S-adenosyl-methionine, naproxen and placebo in the treatment of degenerative joint disease. Am J Med 83 (Suppl 5A):66–71, 1987
13. Chabal C, Jacobson L, Chaney EF, et al: Narcotics for chronic pain: Yes and no? A useless dichotomy. American Pain Society Journal, in press
14. Davidoff G, Guarracini M, Roth E, et al: Trazodone hydrochloride in the treatment of dysesthetic pain in traumatic myelopathy: A randomized double blind placebo controlled study. Pain 29:151–161, 1987
15. Devoghel JC: Small intrathecal doses of lysine acetylsalicylate relieve intractable pain in man. J Int Med Res 11:90–91, 1983
16. Ferreira SH, Lorenzetti BB, Correa FMA: Central and peripheral antialgesic action of aspirin-like drugs. Eur J Pharmacol 53:39–48, 1978
17. Flower RJ, Moncada S, Vane JR: Analgesics, antipyretics and anti-inflammatory agents: Drugs used in the treatment of gout. *In* Gilman AG, Goodman, LS, Rall TW, et al (eds): Goodman and Gilman's The Pharmacological Basis of Therapeutics, ed 7. New York, Macmillan, 1985, pp 674–715
18. Fordyce WE: On opioids and treatment targets. American Pain Society Bulletin 1(4):1–4, 1991
19. Frank RG, Kashani JH, Parker JC, et al: Antidepressant analgesia in rheumatoid arthritis. J Rheumatol 15:1632–1638, 1988
20. Ganvir P, Beaumont G, Seldup J: A comparative trial of clomipramine and placebo as adjunctive therapy in arthralgia. J Int Med Res 8:60–66, 1980
21. Goldenberg DL, Felson DT, Dinerman H: A randomized controlled trial of amitriptyline and naproxen in the treatment of patients with fibromyalgia. Arthritis Rheum 29:1371–1377, 1986
22. Gourlay GK, Willis RJ, Wilson PR: Postoperative pain control with methadone: Influence of supplementary methadone doses and blood concentration-response relationships. Anesthesiology 61:19–26, 1984
23. Grace EM, Bellamy N, Kassam Y, et al: Controlled, double-blind, randomized trial of amitriptyline in relieving articular pain and tenderness in patients with rheumatoid arthritis. Curr Med Res Opin 9:426–429, 1985

24. Gringas M: A clinical trial of tofranil in rheumatic pain in general practice. J Int Med Res 4(suppl 2):41–49, 1976
25. Halpern LM: Psychotropic drugs and the management of chronic pain. *In* Bonica JJ (ed): Advances in Neurology. New York, Raven Press, 1975, pp 539–545
26. Hameroff SR, Cork RC, Scherer K, et al: Doxepin effects on chronic pain, depression and plasma levels of opioids. J Clin Psychiatry 43:22–27, 1982
27. Hunskaar S, Fasmer OB, Hole K: Acetylsalicylic acid, paracetamol and morphine inhibit behavioural responses to intrathecally administered substance P or capsaicin. Life Sci 37:1835–1841, 1985
28. Jenkins GD, Ebbutt AF, Evans CD: Tofranil in the treatment of low back pain. J Int Med Res 4(suppl 2):28–40, 1976
29. Kishore-Kumar R, Max MB, Schafer SC, et al: Desipramine relieves post-herpetic neuralgia. Clin Pharmacol Ther 47:305–312, 1990
30. Kjaersgaard-Anderson P, Nafei A, Skov O, et al: Codeine plus paracetamol versus paracetamol in longer-term treatment of chronic pain due to osteoarthritis of the hip: A randomised, double-blind, multi-centre study. Pain 43:309–318, 1990
31. Kvinesdal B, Molin J, Froland A, et al: Imipramine treatment of painful diabetic neuropathy. JAMA 251:1727–1730, 1984
32. Lasagna L, Prescott LF (eds): Non-narcotic analgesics today: Benefits and risks. Drugs 32(suppl 4):1–208, 1986
33. Leijon G, Boivie J: Central post stroke pain: A controlled trial of amitriptyline and carbamazepine. Pain 36:27–36, 1989
34. Lim RK, Guzman F, Rodgers DW, et al: Site on action of narcotic and nonnarcotic analgesics determined by blocking bradykinin evoked visceral pain. Arch Int Pharmacodyn Ther 152:25–58, 1964
35. Loeser JD: Concepts of pain. *In* Stanton-Hicks M, Boas R (eds): Chronic Low Back Pain. New York, Raven Press, 1982, p 146
36. Magni G: The use of antidepressants in the treatment of chronic pain. Drugs 42:730–748, 1991
37. Maruta T, Swanson DW: Problems with the use of oxycodone compound in patients with chronic pain. Pain 11:389–396, 1981
38. Maruta T, Swanson DW, Finlayson RE: Drug use and dependency in patients with chronic pain. Mayo Clin Proc 54:241–244, 1979
39. Max MB, Culnane M, Schafer SC, et al: Amitriptyline relieves diabetic neuropathy pain in patients with normal or depressed mood. Neurology 37:589–596, 1987
40. Max MB, Kishore-Kumar R, Schafer SC, et al: Efficacy of desipramine in painful diabetic neuropathy: A placebo controlled trial. Pain 45:3–9, 1991
41. Max MB, Lynch SA, Muir J, et al: Effects of desipramine, amitriptyline and fluoxetine on pain in diabetic neuropathy. N Engl J Med 326:1250–1256, 1992
42. McQuay HJ: Pharmacologic treatment of neuralgic and neuropathic pain. Cancer 7:141–159, 1988
43. Monks R: Psychotropic drugs. *In* Bonica JJ (ed): The Management of Pain, ed 2. Philadelphia, Lea and Febiger, 1990, pp 1676–1689
44. Pheasant H, Bursk A, Goldfarb J, et al: Amitriptyline and chronic low back pain: A randomized double blind cross over study. Spine 8:552–557, 1983
45. Piletta P, Porchet HC, Dayer P: Distinct central nervous system involvement of paracetamol and salicylate. *In* Bond MR, Charlton JE, Woolf CJ (eds): Proceedings of the VI World Congress on Pain. New York, Elsevier, 1991, pp 181–184
46. Portenoy RK: Chronic opioid therapy for non malignant pain. Journal of Pain and Symptom Management 5:S46–62, 1990
47. Portenoy RK: Chronic opioid therapy for persistent noncancer pain: Can we get past the bias? American Pain Society Bulletin 1(2):1–5, 1991
48. Portenoy RK: Opioid therapy for chronic noncancer pain: The issue revisited. American Pain Society Bulletin 1(4):4–7, 1991
49. Portenoy RK, Foley KM: Chronic use of opioid analgesics in non-malignant pain. Pain 25:171–186, 1986
50. Porter J, Jick H: Addiction rare in patients treated with narcotics. N Engl J Med 302:123–128, 1980

51. Ramwell PW, Shaw JE, Jessup R: Spontaneous and evoked release of prostaglandins from frog spinal cord. Am J Physiol 211:998–1004, 1966
52. Sarzi Puttini P, Cazzola M, Bocassini L, et al: A comparison of dothiepin versus placebo in the treatment of pain in rheumatoid arthritis and the association of pain with depression. J Int Med Res 16:331–337, 1988
53. Sindrup SH, Ejlertsen B, Froland A, et al: Imipramine treatment in diabetic neuropathy relief of subjective symptoms without changes in peripheral and autonomic nerve function. Eur J Clin Pharmacol 37:151–153, 1989
54. Staples JS, Buckley FP: Opioid and sedative/tranquilliser consumption in outpatients with chronic non malignant pain. Clinical Journal of Pain, in press
55. Taiwo YO, Levine JD: Prostaglandins inhibit endogenous pain control mechanisms by blocking transmission at spinal noradrenergic synapses. J Neurosci 8:1346–1349, 1988
56. Taub A: Opioid analgesics in the treatment of chronic intractable pain of non-neoplastic origin. *In* Kitshata LM (ed): Narcotic Analgesics in Anesthesiology. Baltimore, Williams & Wilkins, 1982, pp 199–208
57. Tavoni A, Vitali C, Bombardieri S, et al: Evaluation of S-adenasy-methionine in primary fibromyalgia: A double-blind cross over study. Am J Med 83(suppl 5A):107–110, 1987
58. Tennant FS, Uelman GF: Narcotic maintenance for chronic pain: Medical and legal guidelines. Postgrad Med J 73:81–94, 1983
59. Tennant FS, Robinson D, Sagahrian A, et al: Chronic opioid treatment of intractable non-malignant pain. Pain Management (Jan/Feb):18–36, 1988
60. Tennant FS, Rawson RA: Outpatient treatment of prescription opioid dependence: Comparison of two methods. Arch Intern Med 142:1845–1847, 1982
61. Thorpe P, Marchant-Williams R: The role of an antidepressant, dibenzepine, in the relief of pain in chronic arthritic states. Med J Aust 1:264–266, 1974
62. Turk DC, Brodie MC: Chronic opioid therapy for persistent non cancer pain: Panacea or oxymoron? American Pain Society Bulletin 1(1):1–6, 1991
63. Turner JA, Calsyn DA, Fordyce WE, et al: Drug utilization patterns in chronic pain patients. Pain 8:357–363, 1982
64. Urban BJ, France RD, Steinberger DL, et al: Long term use of narcotic/antidepressant medication in the management of phantom limb pain. Pain 24:191–197, 1986
65. Ward NG: Tricyclic antidepressants for chronic low back pain: Mechanisms of action and predictors of response. Spine 11:661–665, 1986
66. Watson CP, Evans RJ, Reed K, et al: Amitriptyline versus placebo in post-herpetic neuralgia. Neurology 32:671–673, 1982
67. Willer J-C, De Broucker T, Bussel B, et al: Central analgesic effect of ketoprofen in humans: Electrophysiologic evidence for a supraspinal mechanism in a double-blind cross over study. Pain 38:1–7, 1989
68. Yaksh TL: Central and peripheral mechanisms for the antialgesic action of acetylsalicylic acid. *In* Barnett HJM, Hurst JU, Mustard JF (eds): Acetylsalicylic Acid: New Uses for an Old Drug. New York, Raven Press, 1982, pp 137–151
69. Zenz M, Strumpf M, Tryba M: Long term oral opioid therapy in patients with chronic nonmalignant pain. Journal of Pain and Symptom Management 7:69–77, 1992

Address reprint requests to

F. Peter Buckley, MB, FFARCS
Pain and Toxicity Program, FB600
Fred Hutchinson Cancer Research Center
1124 Columbia Street
Seattle, WA 98104

PRESCRIPTION OF REHABILITATION REGIMENS IN THE MANAGEMENT OF PAIN

Mark A. Tomski, MD, and Thomas B. Corsolini, PT, MD

There is a paucity of literature regarding the physician's role in the prescription of rehabilitation regimens in the management of the patient with pain syndromes.[1, 2, 3] Despite the lack of guidance from the literature, any physician treating patients with complaints of pain is likely to make use of physical therapy and occupational therapy, usually on a frequent basis, and psychological services may also be requested.

Currently, in most states, only a licensed physician may write for prescription of therapy treatments (physical therapy and occupational therapy). In some states, physical and occupational therapists are allowed by law to evaluate and prescribe programs independently of physicians. Despite the advent of direct access, third-party payers still recognize and value the medical diagnosis and frequently pay for therapy services only when they are prescribed by a licensed physician.

All too frequently, physicians have often given little thought to prescribing of these services; however, heightened scrutiny will bring pressure on physicians to be precise and goal oriented when ordering allied health care services.

The physician's role in the prescription and monitoring of therapy services has recently been questioned. Stanton et al,[5] in a survey of resident physicians, found that there was a deficit in resident physicians' knowledge of physical therapy, as measured by a questionnaire, despite these same physicians' feeling adequately informed (prepared) to prescribe such therapy. In addition, some therapists are redefining their own "physical therapy diagnosis."

From the University of Washington, Seattle (MAT); and private practice, Corvallis, Oregon (TBC)

Sahrmann[4] has proposed the following definition of physical therapy diagnosis:

Diagnosis is the term that names the primary dysfunction toward which the physical therapist directs treatment. The dysfunction is identified by the physical therapist based on information obtained from the history, signs, symptoms, examination, and tests the therapist performs or requests.

The aforementioned examples strongly support the physician's need to be active in the prescription, direction, and monitoring of all therapy services. *Dorland's Illustrated Medical Dictionary*, 27th edition, defines diagnosis as "the art of distinguishing one disease from another." Diagnosis in this context requires a complete understanding of the patient's disease state and its pathophysiology, associated functional limitations, and natural history. Another study, by Uili et al,[6] found that both physicians in practice for 10 years or longer and physiatrists had adequate knowledge of physical-therapy procedures. If a physician is unclear as to the appropriateness or the adequate dosage and monitoring of the therapy regimen, a referral to a specialist is in order, rather than abdication of the physician's responsibility for total patient care to a limited practitioner.

Therapy regimens can be divided into three aspects: (1) passive measures, (2) active measures, and (3) educational measures. Passive measures are physical agents such as heat, electricity, and massage, in which the patient plays no active role. Passive therapies generally are helpful in initiating and preparing patients for more active therapy or for pain relief in the acute phase.

Active therapies are primarily strengthening, endurance, and aerobic exercise regimens that are monitored and prescribed by the therapists.

Education can be in specific home regimens, energy conversion techniques, body mechanics, and the like. Included under this rubric are behavioral strategies to improve patient performance in physical and home programs (e.g., graphs, charts, encouragement and other positive reinforcers of patient performance).

When prescribing therapies, the physician should keep in mind which specific areas he or she would like the therapy regimen to include.

THERAPY PRESCRIPTION

In writing for therapy regimens in managing patients with pain, the use of therapy checklists should be avoided. Written individualized prescriptions facilitate the thinking process and result in a better prescription. There are six basic elements in the prescription of therapy: (1) medical diagnosis, (2) precautions, (3) goals, (4) type of therapy, (5) frequency and duration, and (6) physician recheck.

The medical diagnosis should be as specific as possible and should avoid merely stating the condition of pain, such as "shoulder pain" or "low back pain." The more specific the diagnosis, the more helpful to the therapists and the greater chance for successful treatment.

Precautions are essential in giving directions to the therapists and include weight-bearing status, limitations of range of motion, cardiac precautions, use of no deep heat in malignancy, avoidance of ultrasound in pregnancy, and so on.

Goals should be conceptualized along the lines of thinking in terms of passive, active, and educative types of therapy. Pain reduction alone should never be the goal of therapy. Use of modalities for pain reduction, active exercises for strength and endurance, and education for knowledge of body mechanics and injury prevention are examples of appropriate goals in the management of pain.

Frequency and duration of the therapy regimen should be monitored closely by the physician. Early in the treatment of the patient, the frequency may be high and gradually spread out, with the eventual prescription of a home regimen when the specific goals have been met.

The return to the physician for recheck should be included in the prescription so the therapist(s) will know when to have the therapy evaluation and progress notes available to the physician for review at the patient's follow-up visit.

It is essential that the physician and the therapist maintain an open dialogue, because the physician has knowledge that the therapist does not have, and vice versa, especially with respect to patient's response to treatment.

With the aforementioned format in mind, there is no room in prescribing the all too common "evaluate and treat" in managing the patient with pain with a therapy regimen. "Evaluate and treat" is analogous to sending of a pharmaceutical prescription of "please give 'heart pill' " in a case of congestive heart failure.

SUMMARY

In summary, the prescription of rehabilitation regimens and the management of the patient with pain are activities that should not be taken lightly by physicians. Physicians are responsible for monitoring response to treatment and progress toward goals in determining the duration of treatment. It is important for the physician to leave open doors of communication between the therapist, the patient, and himself or herself. The goals are optimal management of the patient, with reduction of pain and return to their previous role, improved function, or maximal functional improvement while using limited resources most efficiently.

References

1. Currie DM, Margurger RA: Writing therapy referrals and treatment plans and the interdisciplinary team. *In* DeLisa JA (ed): Rehabilitation Medicine. Philadelphia, JB Lippincott, 1988
2. Martin GM: Prescribing physical and occupational therapy. *In* Kottke FJ, Stillwell GK, Lehmann JF (eds): Krusen's Handbook of Physical Medicine and Rehabilitation. Philadelphia, WB Saunders, 1982
3. Prescription of therapy. *In* Okamoto GA (ed): Physical Medicine and Rehabilitation. Philadelphia, WB Saunders, 1984
4. Sahrmann SA: Diagnosis by the physical therapist—a prerequisite for treatment: A special communication. Phys Ther 68:1703–1706, 1988
5. Stanton PE, Fox FK, Frangos KM, et al: Assessment of resident physicians' knowledge of physical therapy. Phys Ther 65:27–30, 1985
6. Uili RM, Shepard KF, Savinar E: Physician knowledge and utilization of physical therapy procedures. Phys Ther 64:1523–1530, 1984

Address reprint requests to

Mark A. Tomski, MD
7329 18th Avenue NW
Seattle, WA 98117

1047–9651/93 $0.00 + .20

A DEFINITION AND APPROACH TO HELPING THE PATIENT WITH A RETURN-TO-WORK PREDICAMENT

Stanley J. Bigos, MD, Randy Baker, RA, and Sid Lee, RA

THE AMERICAN RETURN-TO-WORK PREDICAMENT

Henry Ford, Andrew Carnegie, John Rockefeller, and other visionaries, through the corporate organization of the manufacturing revolution, built a strong middle class in America.[8] The wages they paid increased the opportunity for hourly workers then to buy their cheaper mass-produced products. One result of this revolution was the improved chance for an uneducated worker to reach a middle-class standard of living. Mass production and expansion of the middle class created the greatest market for goods that the world has known.

The system worked remarkably well until it had to face international competition. When American industries competed only among themselves for this expanding market, there was at least a national balance, with the fruits of the winners balancing the spoils of the losers. Workers still lost their jobs from national competition, but the shifts of opportunity were to a neighboring locale. Gradually, however, our markets became the target of industries beyond our borders. Then, losses to international competitors provided neither regional nor national compensatory mechanisms. Lost jobs from international competition expanded the pool of workers competing for the fewer remaining jobs and drove down wages. The effect has been not only an erosion of the middle class built during the manufacturing revolution but a concurrent and significant effect on the livelihood of those with less education and fewer skills. More succinctly, the loss of jobs especially affects those who, in the absence of a manufacturing base, have fewer job opportunities when they can no longer use their musculoskeletal system as a crane. This may well be the link between our transition from being the

From the Department of Orthopaedics, University of Washington, Seattle, Washington (SJB, RB); and UCLA Emergency Medical Center, Los Angeles, California (SL)

---

manufacturing giant of the world to a service community over a 20-year period from 1960 to 1980 with a parallel increase (2700%) in back pain disability awards by the Social Security Administration.[22, 28]

It is difficult to explain the 2700% increase in back pain disability awards solely by changes in injury mechanisms or human physiology. By the 1980s, it was reported that, because of increasing labor costs, the United States could not be a competitive manufacturer any longer despite a decrease in wages. International competition drove relative wages down by reducing the number of available jobs and increasing the pool of available American workers.[26, 27] Whether cause or effect, the greatest expansion in labor costs has been in benefits.[16] In combination with this expense has been the growth of an adversarial insurance service system to deal with workplace injuries, especially the most expensive one, related to back problems.

The development of this system can, at least in part, be attributed to the nature of back pain itself. Back problems are common and seem to be an unavoidable part of life, affecting virtually everyone before retirement age[17] (Holtman G: personal communication). The diagnostic criteria for the physiologic or inciting cause of back symptoms are often confusing and difficult to discern. The confusion is compounded when this inevitable part of life is considered a compensable injury for industrial insurance purposes. The creation of the term *industrial back pain* apparently fostered the development of adversarial attitudes and expensive systems that have only worsened the burden by expanding costs without returning the injured worker to productivity. "Adversarial help" seems, and mostly is, a contradiction in terms. In any event, this "adversarial help" system, although a growing expense, has had little effect in aiding either the worker or society by reaching the goal of keeping our populace productive until retirement age.

By the early 1980s labor costs were said to be so great, despite decreasing relative wages,[26, 27] that all manufacturing was destined only for Third World countries.[2, 3, 9] Yet today, Japan and Germany, which have a higher standard of living than ours, also stand as the major worldwide manufacturers and exporters.[19, 34] What makes them different? The societal pressures and differences between Japan and the United States are complex, but the German social mores are less dissimilar. Data indicate that in Germany, worker productivity and hours worked per week are lower than in the United States but wages are actually higher.[16] Yet, in 1986, West Germany's exports exceeded those of the much larger United States of America.[19] One reason that has been entertained is that the cost for back pain alone in West Germany was only one tenth to one twelfth per worker than in genetically similar countries such as Sweden.[17] Could this be related to the fact that in Germany, back pain is not considered a compensable, disabling injury?

The German worker security system originated in the 1870s, when back pain was still considered to be an expected part of life.[10] It provides workers with gradually decreasing time-loss but not a disability award to be fought over by expensive insurance personnel, evaluating physicians, and attorneys. How, then, does their system deal with workers who lose their capacity for heavy labor? First, the Germans have seemed more guild- and apprenticeship-oriented, with heavier work carried out by younger members. Second, in the 1960s they also established the Berufsgenossenschaftsverband law to subsidize worker retraining. This law was passed to provide credit toward retraining later in life for each year worked at hourly jobs. The more years an individual worked, the more money was in this fund for his or her use for retraining. This fund has been available at the worker's discretion. Thus, if a worker has a back problem or any other age-related problem that interferes with work, he or she receives gradually decreasing time-loss as wage replacement. Being in control, the worker has the option to retrain or return to work, depending on the amount of retraining credit that he or she has accumulated in the fund. At first this may seem like an expensive program, but the potential for economic impact on their system is obvious: (1) It eliminates the administrative cost of expensive insurance personnel, attorneys, and physicians needed in our system to argue over potential disability money; (2) it empowers the worker; and (3) perhaps it relieves some of the uncertainties felt by investors about potential future employee costs and liabilities related to any manufacturing. The situation seems markedly different on all three points in the United States at this time.

Comparatively, the injured American worker faces an adversarial system. The defensive posturing on both sides seems to stem from confusion that occurs because back pain is considered an injury. Safety-program demands such as "don't hurt your back" and the patient's response that "they did this to me" illustrate adversarial attitudes that may be present long before back pain occurs. The workers' understanding of insurance in this system for these types of injury may be quite different from reality. This "adversarial worker insurance" system is really an "employer cost assurance" program to help set production costs by assuring the cost of industrial injuries for the next fiscal period. Insurance/assurance systems tend to be geared more toward the management of money than to helping workers who become patients. The system is rewarded for the accuracy of predicting future costs and is allowed to gain interest from the escrow money being managed. Thus, this insurance/assurance system benefits from holding money early in the fiscal period (when there is more money in the coffers to gain interest) and then spending it all at the end of the fiscal period to hit the projected mark accurately. The authors have noted that there are more requests for evaluations, independent medical examinations, and contracts for expensive programs at the end of the fiscal year than at the beginning of the next. Thus, employers are satisfied that costs are accurately projected and they are relieved from having to pay additional costs or tying up more money in escrow than is absolutely necessary.

Those money-management aspects can be exemplified in many ways. One example was brought to my attention by a patient trying to close his claim. He found that his "insurance/assurance company" had not paid $1800 worth of services rendered at my institution over a 3-year period. When asking, he was told that "the University only billed them once," apparently indicating that they respond only after multiple requests.

Consider the short-sightedness illustrated by the experience of one of our patients. One day, he received a call from an irritated state industrial insurance executive accusing him of manipulating the system by becoming the first person to receive 16 months of retraining benefits ($3000) to attend the University of Washington. In anger, he was also assured that he would be the last. This claimant worked mostly as a northwest tree faller until age 38. I first saw him for his second serious back problem and encouraged him to consider what he might be able to do until age 65. Because the majority of northwest tree falling is done as piecework, he knew that $48 per day was always withheld for Industrial Injury Insurance. Thus, he expected some help from this daily donation, totalling more than $250,000, to make a transition after he could not physically continue to work as a tree faller. He described the rude demeanor and intonations that greeted him from the beginning by claims managers. After he attained his high-school equivalency and was found to have an IQ of 176, an industrial-insurance-funded vocational rehabilitation counselor recommended that he needed no training and should get a job as a used-car salesman, but he took it personally on himself to learn the system well enough to get some limited workmens' compensation help through his own tenacity and ingenuity. He completed college in 3 years, mostly on his own resources, maintaining more than a 3.9/4.0 grade point average.

He also studied how the insurance system worked, and using political lobbyists instead of attorneys, he applied external pressure to hold claims managers to the letter of the law rather than to the convenient bureaucratically construed guidelines. This provided him with the educational help for the last 16 months of his schooling, 5 years after his original claim. This came to about $3000 for the 16 months of help for which he was chastised.

The present disability system sometimes seems to lose sight of its goal. Should emotionally charged, talented attorneys in their 20s and 30s waste their abilities and energies voraciously fighting in my office over forcing a 52-year-old fisherman, with two failed back surgeries, to return to a commercial fishing job that none of them at a much younger age could physically tolerate? Should an insurance company argue, through an expensive deposition, about paying a $475 treatment bill that returned an individual to work because they have already spent thousands of dollars on the vocational paper chases, pain clinics, and surgeries that had been unsuccessful? Daily, in my medical practice, I commonly receive calls and information from the insurance company, painting the patient as the culprit. This intended benefit has inadvertently developed into a feudal adversarial system.

The system can also provide employers with a personnel management advantage that hides real motives behind a worker safety role by allowing them to be rid of unwanted employees. For instance, as a physician I commonly hear, "There is no limited duty!," "Union rule!," "Company rule!," and "Can't take them back until they're 100%!" In many instances these rules are invoked only for unwanted employees. Many of my patients verbalize an understanding of an unwritten rule that after a back injury claim or any time loss related to back pain, the chance of being laid off for any reason is markedly increased. Workers who want to keep their jobs may hold out for as long as possible before making a claim, after thinking through the potential impact of their decision. Significant data show that 50% of workers each year have back problems that can interfere with work or recreational activity but only 2% to 5% file a back injury claim.[24, 30, 31] More and more data implicate the influence of nonphysical factors in the report of back problems at work.[4, 5, 29] The decision to file subsequently becomes further emotionalized for the worker with the realization that this industrial insurance/assurance is truly adversarial.

Workers have to deal with the return-to-work predicament, which can be associated with many varied problems. They may not be able physically to do the work any longer. It may also be that they definitely cannot continue to do this particular job until retirement. Probably, and more importantly, these realities combine a feeling of not being wanted with feeling a continuous jeopardy of being laid off with a minimum of comparable benefits. Why do systems provide only enough educational help for someone to become a lawnmower repairman and obstacles toward greater ability or opportunities? Is there something kind about forcing people to be declared disabled as an alternative to facing failure related to being unable to do job tasks until retirement age? Workers do not seem to derive enjoyment from proving how sick they are or subjecting themselves to long periods devoid of the emotional energy related to a sense of achievement or related camaraderie. Should the money subsidizing well-educated insurance company personnel, attorneys, and evaluating physicians not rightfully be going to the workers who usually have earned an opportunity, through the sweat of their original career, to maintain their dignity with a chance to be productive taxpayers until retirement age? It has been argued that some workers would take advantage of such a system, but considering our present ineffectiveness, could any do so to the extent of us professionals in the disability network? Few of us could win that argument. Perhaps the German system of subsidizing worker retraining rather than disability-producing professionals is more than a reasonable alternative.

Data in the literature indicate that our adversarial approach is inherently harmful to workers trapped in this system.[12] Under stress, individuals seem to regress and commonly concentrate their focus on the back pain as the source of all their problems. Who would not feel threatened by an adversarial system that is trying to force him or her to face failure? It is important to realize how emotional this threatened state of mind can be. Primary prevention must begin with changing the adversarial system and attitudes that do nothing to reduce the emotionalization of the problem or curb the frustration of caring medically for insured workers.

THE INDIVIDUAL PREDICAMENT

There are fewer options for those individuals who do not have a college education to change occupations when they can no longer use their back in strenuous jobs. They could toughen up for a few more years before facing an inevitable change in occupations, but career changing options tend not to improve with age, especially after yet another injury claim. We may see them as needing to go back to school, but who is to say that workers will be less intimidated than they were after high school when originally deciding against further education? It is also important to realize that our population, when compared with their German counterparts, has a lesser chance of being literate enough to return to school, and there are significant school-related costs that are not a barrier in other countries. Another comparable distinction is that health care is automatically available for the German worker's family while retraining is being accomplished. Although we do have retraining options for workers, in reality most do not qualify until depleted of emotional energy and dignity over the year or more needed to prove to an adversarial system that they are disabled enough to be allowed to retrain in the cheapest program available. Their only other option is to find another hourly job that can be tolerated until age 65. Today, however, there are fewer opportunities in our service-oriented society for someone without a college degree who can no longer use his or her musculoskeletal system as a crane, compared with when we were more of a manufacturing society.

All these factors contribute to the lumbar spine as the site of a most expensive health care problem in the 20-to-50 age group, the most expensive industrial injury, by far the most expensive musculoskeletal problem, and the most common cause of disability in those under age 45.[15, 18, 24] For the thoughtful health care provider, back pain has become most frustrating, and in recent years this frustration is spreading to other age-related problems now considered injuries for insurance company purposes.

What can the thoughtful health care provider do to make a difference and to help? If the patient does not respond rapidly to the care we provide, take, at most, 4 minutes from being a doctor and try the role of being a friend to your patient. This method not only saves time and frustration but may actually make a difference.

This process seemed difficult to me until I realized how insidiously certain attitudes develop. A young Danish physician recently enlightened me to what is not always obvious. This former Falster Island farm boy practiced in northern

Scandinavia immediately after finishing medical school. In this rural setting, he saw patients and was delighted by the interesting personal stories most of them had to tell. He noticed a similar delight when first beginning work in a back center in Copenhagen among patients trying a new back treatment program. He was struck, however, by the contrast with patients ordered to go there by the insurance company.

He sensed these patients to be frustrated by both their own situation and the insurance system. Their cautious attitude did not allow them to divulge their story as many of his northern Scandinavian patients had done. He was also struck by his own growing frustration, sensing the distrust and the potential for his personal failure as a physician. But his unique background, perhaps being young in his career and wise enough to understand himself, exposed an uneasiness toward settling into his role in an adversarial system by focusing his frustrations on patients commonly labelled "shirker" or "system-beater" by the insurance company. It was enlightening as he related his inability to find within the Hippocratic oath a phrase that suggested doctors should add to a person's burden for the sin of losing a job, resenting the adversarial climate, or not wanting to go through physical discomfort made pointless as soon as benefits are cut off and they are forced to join the 10% already unemployed in Denmark. Is this what caring for the patient has come to, just because the nonphysical factors commonly combine with the physical to interfere with our patient's ability to respond to our treatment and care? Perhaps our blind spots do complicate how we respond as providers to our patients' return to work predicament.

It now goes without saying that non-physical factors can significantly influence the patient's response, not only to back symptoms but to the treatment we provide.[4, 14, 23, 35] Prospective data indicate that not enjoying job tasks and distress in life do affect industrial back problems.[4, 5] In the industrial setting, the relation of back symptoms to back injury claim seems to be more like the proverbial last straw that breaks the back of the already overburdened camel. From that treatment standpoint, there is no biomechanician who would expect the removal only of the last straw to spring the downed camel back to his feet. It becomes obvious that if back pain is that last straw, concentrating strictly on physical treatment but ignoring the other burdens does not always return the injured worker to his feet, to his station in life, or back to work. The following guidelines recognize these nonphysical influences through the patient's response to our treatment recommendations. It also helps us avoid some of the frustrations common in caring for the industrially injured worker by giving timely recommendations to deal with the inevitable or at least by giving reassurance to the patient that we have his or her interests in mind.

It is not practical to surmise that nonphysical factors alone cause musculoskeletal problems. Many age-related problems such as back pain are expected yearly in 50% of working age people,[30, 31] but only 2% to 5% file a back injury claim.[24] A growing body of data now objectifies what Nortin Hadler described as the "return to work predicament," which, even more than the pathology, can affect the outcome.[13] The following guidelines should help in the recognition of nonphysical factors that may interfere with the patient's response to treatment and, more importantly, avoid recrimination and undue frustration.

EARLY HINTS OF A RETURN-TO-WORK PREDICAMENT

The influence of nonphysical factors slowing or blocking recovery may be recognizable in the initial patient history and physical examination as inconsistencies, emphasis on suffering (rather than symptoms), in back pain with more than two of five positive Waddell tests, or abnormal pain drawings.[20, 23, 33] Although the descriptions of physical symptoms tend to be localized, descriptions of suffering tend to be vague, with an emphasis on intensity. It is important to recognize that recording inconsistencies and symptom embellishment in the acute patient have not provided us with useful labels for diagnosing or treating these patients.

Do not regard such pain-magnifying behavior as an indication of malingering, which can rarely be proven. No purpose is served by a physician's questioning the patient's integrity. Raising the issue of malingering diminishes cooperation and benefits only the attorneys who might profit monetarily from a stronger adversarial stance.

Pain behavior is but a higher level of the behavioral changes observed in a threatened animal. These patients may feel "trapped" and without options in a system in which everyone seems to be trying to force them to face failure. The feeling of failure may be totally related to the physical symptoms in a physically strenuous job, or partially related in a less strenuous job that has exhausted their intellectual, energy, or personality capacities. Such pain behavior is most constructively interpreted as a way of asking for help from the physician, whom the patient hopes has his or her best interest in mind. Thus, it is very important to avoid being perceived as acting on the behalf of the insurance company or the employer.

Although pain embellishments can become ingrained behavior in the more chronic patient it is safer to assume that in the acute patient they are distress signals. Pain behavior that continues at a high level after 4 to 6 weeks of care probably indicates that the patient is not convinced that we truly have his or her best interest in mind. Pain behavior provides an index of suspicion that nonphysical pressures may slow recovery and are best dealt with by actively monitoring the patient's response to a series of helpful recommendations. This approach can be time efficient and less recriminating when one is dealing with potentially sensitive issues by projecting honestly to the patient that you are truly there to help, not to judge.

MONITORING THE PATIENT'S PROGRESS

A history and physical examination generally lead to recommendations for symptom control, with a reassuring explanation about the medical problem. We then modify activity to the needs of the patient, first to avoid debilitation and then to provide protective muscular conditioning. Because nonphysical pressures are often difficult to define early in treatment, monitoring the patient's response to our recommendations and taking appropriate action keep us on track so we can provide the most effective, timely help. Unfortunately, the success of our treatment in our complex society is not always accomplished through physical recommendations or procedures alone. We first approach the back-to-work predicament either when asked about work restrictions or when the response to physical conditioning is inadequate for return to full duty.

Humane, Reasonable Limitations

Early physical restrictions are an application of known back biomechanics to the patient's estimate of physical limitations. We can stress goals and warn patients that the maximal time we can recommend for each level of limitation is intended to allow ample time for protective muscular retraining. We can also emphasize that restrictions are time limited, not for protection but to help control symptoms during muscular conditioning. Many difficulties encountered with this approach are more likely associated with the return-to-work predicament than the physical pathology.

Because our treatment is commonly expected to return the worker to the work site, the medical profession has developed some rather harsh methods to accomplish this goal. Work or ability hardening, as a concept, pushes the medical model toward overcoming the nonphysical factors. The original idea was to encourage patients and help them overcome their fears by proving that they can safely use their back. Taken to the extreme, some insurance systems use this approach as a behavior modification campaign to make it more physically demanding to be sick than to be well enough to return to work. However, many patients are seemingly overcome by their predicament. These workers often must perform their reconditioning programs in a gymnasium and are not allowed to return to work until they are "100%," a common request that serves as an early hint of the severity of the predicament. A more reasonable approach for the patient is to gradually increase the type of activity required at the work site, not at the gymnasium.

Ability hardening programs in the medical setting are usually approached after severe pathology has been ruled out, and the discussion of discomfort is limited as much as possible. The activities blocking return to work are identified and followed by a recording of the patient's attempts to perform specific activities. Then, the patient is "toughened" into an activity by starting out at perhaps half the weight and two thirds of the repetitions for a few sets per day, gradually increasing each aspect until it becomes mechanically more stressful on the back to be off work but working at this treatment program than it is working at the original job tasks. Sometimes, this treatment results in weeks of what patients describe as torture before the insurance company closes their claim.

The Career Decision

To avoid such a scenario, we attempt to approach the predicament before it becomes chronic. If the patient has experienced 4 to 6 weeks of continuous symptoms, we evaluate the patient's bone, joint, nerve, and general health status for potential physical reasons that may be delaying the normal expected recovery. By this time, considerations for surgical intervention should be completed. If the findings lead to surgery or the patient has not been able to return to work, I express my concern for the patient's future. I offer to do anything I can "to save your job if it is something you honestly think you will do until age 65." If the patient cannot recondition sufficiently to return to required duties or if limited duty is not available, the patient must be asked, "Do you think you will be able to do this job there until retirement?" or he or she must question himself or herself, "Do you think they will want you until then?" Patients who cannot answer with positive certainty need to explore career options by gathering enough information to interact effectively with the employer or insurance company. Patients sometimes must be convinced that leaving this important step to someone else rarely leads to a worthwhile outcome (Table 1).

Medical providers can adopt a compassionate approach to the patient's work predicament but must avoid falling into the trap of trying to take away all the pain, figuring out the exact cause of pain, or making the back as good as new. All

Table 1. GUIDE TO APPROACHING THE PREDICAMENT (30 seconds)

Want job or wanted at job until age 65?
1. "I am concerned about your future."
2. "I am willing to help in any way I can to save your job if that is something you plan to do until age 65. I will use all of my influence to secure your job even by calling your employer personally.
   "If the job is not what you think you will do until age 65, figure out your options as soon as possible. You now have extra time, and the more you know, the better the decisions you can make now or later."

Important
1. "Do not wait for the insurance company or employer to decide what will make you happy. Get the information yourself and know your options."
2. "Start a spiral notebook!" (See Table 2, Action IV)

three may be impossible for many of our patients. This approach allows the physician to take the time to be concerned, compassionate, and nonjudgmental, offering to help the patient avoid a personal financial disaster. The worker may be better able to recognize the predicament after attempting physical conditioning and receiving the results of the work-up. The patient must come to understand the need to make a decision about the future, either now, with some assets and your help, or later, alone, after the claim is closed.

Patients stuck in anger because the system is unfair sometimes believe that symptoms are not their fault and it is the responsibility of the insurance company or the employer to provide options. Unfortunately, to win the battle of proving that somebody injured them usually takes years, commonly has a very poor benefit-to-cost ratio, and further burdens the worker with a "loser" label that can haunt the rest of their life. If he or she waits for the employer or insurance company to figure out what will make a worker happy for the rest of his or her life, he or she may be long since retired before it happens. It is important for workers to gather the information on future career options early, because the passing time only lessens the chance for success. Recommendations for gathering information in an organized manner using a spiral notebook are offered in the guidelines described in Table 2. The whole discussion usually takes about 1 minute.

Spiral Notebook

The guidelines for gathering information listed in Table 2 are intended to help patients get beyond the emotional block of not knowing; they must explore their career options to make sound decisions, whether about a different career or staying with their present job. Ask the patient to staple the guidelines into a spiral notebook in which they record their inquiries, bringing it to the clinic for review on each visit. The process requires little physician time and provides two major benefits. First, about 25% of patients quickly and efficiently figure out their options, but half require more coaxing. Medical treatment becomes easier and more successful because less time is spent on symptom embellishment. Patients also tend to make decisions once they have some information. Some feel better about returning to the same job and are more willing to undergo physical conditioning. Others may choose a different career that may or may not require schooling. Most important, the process seems to energize many patients while

Table 2. SPIRAL NOTEBOOK GUIDELINES

Staple this paper inside the cover of a spiral notebook. Use at least one page for each phone call so that they can be grouped later. To figure out what will be best for you in the future, you need information. There are four phases of collecting the information you need to consider.

I. Agencies that can help
   A. Call community colleges for an interview.
      1. Explain your situation.
      2. Ask for recommendations about occupational opportunities and their needed skills.
      3. List phone numbers of potential employers.
   B. Call the Division of Vocational Rehabilitation.
      1. Tell them your situation.
      2. Ask them to send information/interview.
      3. Ask for names of employers who hire for what's hot in your community.
      4. List phone numbers of potential employers.
   C. Consider using career centers (libraries) for same purposes.
II. Call employers in your community or where you want to live.
   A. Ask for names of some of the people who do the job that might interest you.
   B. List phone numbers of employees.
III. Call employees doing what might interest you.
   A. Income?
   B. Toughest part of job?
   C. Recommendations for starting a future in this area in your situation
      1. Training potential
      2. Financial Assistance (How they did it)
      3. Considerations
         a. Present
         b. Future
      4. Ask for the names and numbers of others to contact (same job).
IV. Make 3 × 5 review cards of areas of interest and discuss them with community college advisor/DVR (if available).
   A. Ask for their recommendations.
      1. Preparation
      2. Financial assistance (nondisability)
      3. Full-time/part-time training
   B. Look into financial aspects as recommended and make a budget.

reducing both pain complaints and the physician time spent wrestling with suffering behavior (Table 2).

Dysfunctional Human Behavior

"Behavior is dysfunctional when the haunts of yesterday and fears of tomorrow stand in the way of taking your needs today."

The second benefit of monitoring the career option notebook is to detect how overwhelmed the patient is by the work predicament as depicted by little or no career option activity. Medical treatment is rarely successful while confusion reigns. If the patient fails to create a notebook, point out how uncommon it is for symptoms alone to prevent gathering information by telephone that may be important to the rest of the person's life. A counselor can then be recommended, not for analysis but simply to sort through the areas that might be complicating the patient's recovery and return to work. This process elucidates one of four problems: (1) illiteracy, (2) depression, (3) addiction, or (4) significant dysfunctional behavior (e.g., adult child of alcoholics, preaddiction, depression). The counselor, thereafter, may then support the exploration of career options (Table 3). Usually, a counselor is not required. When the patient begins to believe that you have their best interest in mind, he or she will at that point usually respond with a catharsis. The approach must be similar to that used when approaching an alcoholic. Until he or she realizes they have a problem, any question about alcohol abuse causes a response that is defensive or worse. Only when an excuse for failure is required will the abuser be open to recognizing the real problem related to these dysfunctional elements.

Illiterate patients can be directed to programs that will help them overcome this roadblock to other career options. Depression usually can be treated in conjunction with further physical treatment. Those who have addiction problems while off work tend to increase their habitual use and also experience heightened fears of detection. Addiction needs to be addressed before continuing physical treatment beyond the work-up and acute treatment phases.

Thereafter, communication and understanding need to be established among parties involved with the medical and the work predicament. If needed, a united front can be formed by medical providers, claims manager, perhaps a counselor or support group sponsor (Alcoholics Anonymous, Narcotics Anonymous, Adult Children of Alcoholics, Adult Children Anonymous, union representative) to keep everyone abreast of reasonable time lines for treatment, activity limitations, and stages of exploring the career options.

It is very important to understand that both chronic-pain and acute-pain patients deserve our best recommendations for dealing with the physical problem and the work predicament. With the chronic-pain patients, however, the expectations of a good response are considerably lower. First, many are physically and emotionally debilitated and have more difficulty carrying out the physi-

Table 3. GUIDE TO THE DYSFUNCTIONAL PATIENT (30 seconds)

"Musculoskeletal problems alone do not usually bother people such that they cannot gather information (at least by telephone) to consider options for career change. Other problems can complicate and be complicated by back-to-work difficulties."

"I want you to see a counselor to help you sort through what might be adding pressure in your life and to solicit suggestions on how you might deal with pressure better." "Suggestions never hurt."

Need counselor who can address
1. Literacy
2. Depression
3. Addiction (alcohol/drugs)
4. Unexpressed dysfunctional behavior

The United Front for a Primary Care Contract with the Patient (practitioner, insurance company, counselor, sponsor)

Physical treatment:	Phases/unit time, medications
Humane limitations:	Time period negotiated
Career options:	Community college (interview, GED, hot items), career centers (libraries), Division of Vocational Rehabilitation (hot items)
Dysfunctional:	Get the patient a sponsor (AA, NA, ACA/ACOA)

GED = general equivalency degree; AA = Alcoholics Anonymous; NA = Narcotics Anonymous; ACA/ACOA = Association of Children of Alcoholics.

cal aspects of treatment. Second, they seem to carry more fear and less emotional energy with which to face the predicament the longer they are away from a normal environment. Third, the patient has long convinced employer and co-workers that the illness or injury is severe. Any sudden change in status could be a blow to the person's integrity and support systems. Finally, the patient has become isolated from the work environment and has lost opportunities for gaining emotional energy through experiencing camaraderie or accomplishment. Thus, more acute-pain patients have the best chance of success, especially those with the greatest number of options. Individuals who respond best are those who are well educated (it is difficult to make a notebook about career options if you cannot read or write) and who have not yet been drained of emotional energy. Dealing with the work predicament over time depletes the worker's emotional energy resources, especially in an adversarial insurance system in which patients must prove how sick they are to avoid the consequences of failing in their environment.

A pilot study applying these principles by phone to difficult, chronic back-pain patients was performed by Wiegert & Wiegert & Associates, Omaha, NE (personal communication). To qualify for the study, workers had to be off work for more than 3 months and have failed or been rejected by a work hardening program. The career option help was provided by two individuals who drew on backgrounds in human resources, interviewing, and career counseling and applied emotional activation techniques to encourage the individuals to gather information about their work options until retirement. They actively tried to avoid the passive techniques often applied in the usual vocational rehabilitation or social worker roles. The patients were contacted only by telephone over a 2-month period (mean phone time 91 minutes). Multiple calls were made over the 8-week period to encourage data gathering, with the subsequent follow-up aimed at fostering activating emotional energy needed for gathering the information and decision making. These researchers concentrated their interactive techniques into one of four categories: (1) encouragement to rekindle a feeling of camaraderie, (2) information gathering to foster feelings of achievement, (3) channeling resentment toward proving those they resent to be wrong, and (4) use of fear to overcome inactivity by pointing out the dangers of waiting until the claim is closed to figure out career options until retirement age. Results occurred without any physical treatment for their back problem. Of 21 chronic-pain patients who were off work from 3 to 60 months, contacted only by telephone over a 2-month period, 9 were working and 8 were enrolled in previously overlooked educational programs. Four patients did not cooperate, and one of the patients who did cooperate admitted that he was illiterate, but this was not detected by pain clinic or vocational rehabilitation workers in previous evaluations (Table 4).

Some of the findings stress the basic dilemma that relates to education. None of those who had previously been trained beyond high school returned to their previous employer, but 6 of the cooperative 8 who had never been to college returned to their previous employer rather than choosing to find another employer or an educational program. Most important, those 17 who could be encouraged to gather sufficient information to gain a personal understanding of their career options seemed to make their own career decisions easily. No decision was possible, however, for the quintile who were too dysfunctional even to make a few telephone calls to explore the options available to them for reorienting their lives.

For persons in this latter group, it is important to identify which dysfunctional category (usually illiteracy, depression, addiction, or anxiety) is blocking

Table 4. CAREER OPTIONS BY PHONE

	Previously No Education > HS	Previously Education > HS
New job	0	3
RTW	6	0
Education program	2	5
Dysfunctional	3 (1 illiterate)*	2
Total	11	10

21 consecutive patients failed or turned down for work hardening after off work 3 to 60 months. Almost half returned to previous employer after considering their options if not previously educated beyond high school. None returned to previous employer if educated beyond high school.
 * One who did cooperate was found to be illiterate and began a reading program.
RTW = Return to previous employer; HS = high school.
From Bigos SJ: The practitioners guide to the industrial back problem. II. Helping the Patient with the return to work predicament. Seminars in Spine Surgery 4:62, 1992.

action. Those too dysfunctional to move forward immediately with new career goals require communication and coordination by medical providers, a claims manager, and perhaps a counselor or support group sponsor to keep all abreast of reasonable time lines for treatment, activity limitation, and stages of exploring the career options. Support group sponsors are commonly available through Alcoholics Anonymous, Narcotics Anonymous, Adult Children of Alcoholics, Adult Children Anonymous, and unions. Only through appropriate understanding of the predicament in conjunction with medical treatment can there be a worthwhile outcome for the patient, employer, insurance company, physician, and society as a whole.

SUMMARY

There is little evidence that traditional medical treatment alone turns the tide to decrease disability. There are major differences between the presence of symptoms and disability. For most of the world, our most common disabling problems are an expected part of life, with little recordable evidence of significant medical consequences or disability,[1, 32] but in the industrialized countries with complex disability systems, we seem to have definitions of pain and discomfort confused by the complicated agenda of a disability-oriented insurance system. The result is costly for society and, in many cases, a cold, cruel process for workers who commonly feel trapped without options because of their medical problem alone or in combination with other perceived or real inadequacies. Thus, the future hopes for decreasing the disability problems may well pivot on the understanding that, in many cases, physical treatment alone is insufficient to reach the goal of returning the employee to work.

The return-to-work predicament seems to be a growing factor blocking the outcome we intend for our working-age patients. Thus, if recovery is slow, we must encourage the patient to explore career options. This approach evolved not only from the frustration of dealing with patients but from scientific studies compared to observations in the Third World. Increasing data indicate that physical treatment can be complicated by the return-to-work predicament. We have seen the influence of these nonphysical factors in the treatment models[11, 14, 25, 35] as well as in risk-factor projects such as the Boeing Study,[4–7, 29] in which perceptions, poor job satisfaction, and distress in life tend to overshadow physical factors. The lack of success of medical, pain, and physical models alone echoes the point made to me long ago by Wilbert Fordyce, PhD, who stated: "People don't hurt as much if they have something better to do!" The predicament centers many times around those who do not have something better to do. Is it our job to judge and sentence them or to try to help them find something better to do? I hope the answer is obvious.

This work was supported in part by the Spine Resource Clinic, University of Washington, Seattle, Washington.

References

1. Anderson RT: Orthopaedic ethnography in rural Nepal. Med Anthropol 8:46–59, 1984
2. Barnett DF, Schorsch L: Steel: Upheaval in a Basic Industry. Cambridge, Ballinger, 1983
3. Barnett DF, Crandall RW: Up from the Ashes: The Rise of the Steel Minimill in the United States. Washington, DC, The Brookings Institution, 1986
4. Bigos SJ, Battié MC, Fisher LD, et al: A prospective study of work perceptions and psychosocial factors affecting the report of back injury. Spine 16:1–6, 1991
5. Bigos SJ, Battié MC, Fisher LD, et al: A longitudinal, prospective study of industrial back injury reporting. Clin Orthop 279:21–34, 1992
6. Bigos SJ, Spengler DM, Martin N, et al: Back injuries in industry: A retrospective study. II. Injury factors. Spine 11:246–251, 1986
7. Bigos SJ, Spengler DM, Martin N, et al: Back injuries in industry: A retrospective study. III. Employee related factors. Spine 11:252–256, 1986
8. Chandler AD: The Visible Hand: The Managerial Revolution in American Business. Cambridge, Harvard University Press, 1977
9. Competitive Status of the US Steel Industry. Steel Panel, Committee on Technology and International Economic and Trade Issues. Bruce Old, Chairman. Washington, DC, National Academy Press, 1985
10. Crankshaw E: Bismarck. New York, Viking Press, 1981
11. Fordyce WE: A behavioral analysis of interdisciplinary health care delivery. Perspectives in Behavioral Medicare 3:127–132, 1988
12. Guest GH, Drummond PD: Effect of compensation on emotional state and disability in chronic back pain. Pain 48:125–130, 1992
13. Hadler NM: The predicament of backache. J Occup Med 30:449–450, 1988
14. Herron LD, Turner JA, Weiner P: Lumbar disc herniations: The predictive value of the Health Attribution Test (HAT) and the Minnesota Multiphasic Personality Inventory (MMPI). J Spinal Disorders 1:2–8, 1988
15. Kelsey JL, Pastides H, Bisbee GE, et al: Musculoskeletal Disorders: Their Frequency of Occurrence and Their Impact on the Population of the United States. New York, Prodist, 1978, pp 31–36
16. Manufactures and Minerals—Sales and Profits; Productivity; Mineral Supplies. International Manufacturing Productivity and Labor Costs. US Bureau of Labor Statistics. US Labor Department, 1990
17. Nachemson A: Orsaker, diagnostik och behandling. Onti Ryggen, 1991
18. Nachemson AL, Bigos SJ: The low back. In Cruess RL, Rennie WRJ (eds): Adult Orthopaedics, vol 2. New York, Churchill Livingstone, 1984, pp 843–937
19. Phillips K: The Politics of Rich and Poor: Wealth and the American Electorate in the Reagan Aftermath. Cambridge, Harper Perennial, 1990
20. Ransford AO, Cairns D, Mooney V: The pain drawing as an aid to the psychologic evaluation of patients with low-back pain. Spine 1:127–134, 1976
21. Rossi I: Some observations on the continuous casting of steel. Journal of Metals (March):227–228, 1951
22. Social Security Statistical Supplement (1977–79), Sup. Doc. No. HE 3.3/3.979. Washington, DC, Government Printing Office
23. Spengler DM: Low back pain: Assessment and Management. New York, Grune & Stratton, 1982

24. Spengler DM, Bigos SJ, Martin NA, et al: Back injuries in industry: A retrospective study. I. Overview and cost analysis. Spine 11:241–251, 1986
25. Spengler DM, Freeman C, Westbrook R, et al: Low-back pain following lumbar spine procedures: Failure of initial selection? Spine 5:356–360, 1980
26. Tiffany PA: The Decline of American Steel: How Management, Labor, and Government Went Wrong. New York, Oxford University Press, 1988
27. Time Magazine [Milestones]. July 1, 1991, p 68
28. Toffler A: The Third Wave. New York, Bantam Books, 1980
29. Troup JDG, Foreman TK, Baxter CE, et al: The perception of back pain and the role of psychophysical tests of lifting capacity. 1987 Volvo Award in Clinical Sciences. Spine 12:645–657, 1987
30. Vallfors B: Acute, subacute and chronic low back pain: Clinical symptoms, absenteeism and working environment. Scand J Rehab Med Suppl 11:1–98, 1985
31. Vincente PJ: The Nuprin Report: A summary. Part I. American Pain Society Newsletter, 1988
32. Waddell G: A new clinical model for the treatment of low-back pain. Spine 12:632–644, 1987
33. Waddell G, McCulloch JA, Kummel E, et al: Non-organic physical signs in low back pain. Spine 5:117–125, 1980
34. Welford R: Worker motivation, life time employment and codetermination: Lessons from Japan and West Germany for productivity growth. Contemporary Review 257:129–132, 1990
35. Wiltse LL, Rocchio PD: Preoperative tests as predictors of success of chemonucleolysis in the treatment of the low-back syndrome. J Bone Joint Surg [Am] 57:478–483, 1975

Address reprint requests to

Stanley J. Bigos, MD
Department of Orthopaedics, RK-10
University of Washington
Seattle, WA 98195

MANUAL MEDICINE AND THE OFFICE MANAGEMENT OF PAIN SYNDROMES

Jonathan L. Ritson, MD, and Philip E. Greenman, DO, FAAO

Manual medicine is one of the oldest forms of health care. Hippocrates was known to use manual medicine procedures for the treatment of scoliosis and kyphosis. Galen used manual medicine procedures in the treatment of injuries to the cervical spine. During the Middle Ages, manipulation seemed to fall out of the physician's armamentarium, but in the early 1800s interest was rejuvenated by the work of lay "bone setters," who practiced throughout Europe, particularly within the United Kingdom. Later in the 1800s, Andrew Taylor Still, MD, founded osteopathic medicine and included structural diagnosis and manipulative treatment as a major component of this reform school of medicine. In the 1890s D.D. Palmer founded chiropractic, a limited-scope health care system based extensively on manipulative adjustment as the main treatment intervention.

Manual medicine in the orthodox medical community has grown extensively in the twentieth century. The father-and-son physician teams of James and John Mennell and Edgar and James Cyriax contributed to an increase of manipulative diagnosis and treatment in traditional medicine. The International Federation of Manual Medicine currently is represented in more than 20 countries and has an international membership of more than 7000 physician practitioners.

The musculoskeletal system composes 60% of the human organism. Musculoskeletal pain syndromes are responsible for a large portion of visits to the health care delivery system. In these syndromes, not only is the musculoskeletal system involved but, either directly or through reflex mechanisms, many other organ systems may be encompassed. A thorough structural examination assists in the diagnosis of these syndromes, and frequently, manual medicine treatment procedures are effective.

From Northwest Therapy Spine Program, Tacoma, Washington (JLR); and Departments of Biomechanics and Physical Medicine and Rehabilitation, Michigan State University College of Osteopathic Medicine, East Lansing, Michigan (PEG)

PHYSICAL MEDICINE AND REHABILITATION CLINICS OF NORTH AMERICA

SOMATIC DYSFUNCTION

A thorough structural examination, in addition to the usual orthopedic, neurologic, and vascular components of the physical examination, identifies the manipulable lesion. This entity is entitled *somatic dysfunction* and is defined as "impaired or altered function of related components of the somatic/body framework system (skeletal, arthrodial, and myofascial structures); and related vascular, lymphatic and neural elements."[4] When a full physical examination defines somatic dysfunction as a component of the pain syndrome, manipulative treatment can be appropriately prescribed as a primary restorative measure to the musculoskeletal system in addition to appropriate treatment of an underlying medical condition.

MANIPULATION

To many, *manipulation* means a high-velocity, low-amplitude thrust, with associated joint gapping and popping. *Dorland's Medical Dictionary* defines manipulation as "skillful or dextrous treatment by the hand."[2]

The goal of manipulative treatment is to enhance physiologic states to achieve maximal painless movement of the musculoskeletal system in postural balance. In addition to manipulation, many other tools, such as specific exercise programs, may be applied to assist in the correction and maintenance of postural balance.

THE STRUCTURAL DIAGNOSTIC TRIAD

The diagnosis of somatic dysfunction is based on three elements represented by the mnemonic *ART*. *A* stands for asymmetry of form and function of the musculoskeletal system. *R* deals with range of motion, spanning the spectrum of normal to hypermobile to hypomobile. *T* is related to tissue texture abnormality, primarily of the soft tissue elements of the musculoskeletal system.

In testing for range of motion, one identifies barriers to motion, both normal and abnormal. The end point of active range of motion is called the *physiologic barrier*. The end of the passive range of motion is called the *anatomic barrier*. Each of these barriers has a difference in end feel. A restrictive barrier, because of somatic dysfunction, interferes with both the quantity of motion and the quality of the end feel. Restrictive barriers include muscle spasm, articular and periarticular ligamentous tension, edema, fibrosis, and other myofascial tightness. In evaluating motion, the examiner is interested in range, quality of movement during the range, and quality of the end feel.

MODELS OF MANUAL MEDICINE INTERVENTION

The practice of manual medicine is based on various interventional models. Historically, the emphasis of patient care has stressed disturbances within the internal visceral systems, with little attention given to the musculoskeletal system in maintaining and restoring health. Beyond being the "coat rack" for the internal viscera, the musculoskeletal system is the primary machinery of life through which we act out our humanity and individual personalities in idiosyncratic ways of posture and movement that identify us as individuals. Korr states: "We are not a composite of visceral functions, such as peristalsis, secretions, digestion, vasomotion and glomerular filtration, but a continually changing activity of striated muscles, pulling on bony levers, orchestrated by the central nervous system in response to external and internal stimuli and to volition."[21] He proposed a functional model in which visceral function maintains and services the primary machinery by providing the raw material for cellular metabolism, removing metabolic waste products, dissipating heat, controlling the composition of the extracellular environment, and protecting against foreign substances. Rest corrects incongruency between supply and demand, and if unable, illness results. A holistic model encompasses visceral, behavioral, and musculoskeletal influences on the total organism, and each must be addressed. For example, the elderly recent below-knee amputee with congestive heart failure and increasing shortness of breath and fatigue needs reduction in energy expenditure by proper mechanical gait training, behavioral modification for pacing, and medication changes.

Three different models are described to demonstrate the influence of the musculoskeletal system on total body economy and how manipulative treatment can affect any or all of them by different mechanisms.

Postural/Structural Model

The postural/structural model is one of the most popular used by manual medicine practitioners. It emphasizes the structural relation of the osseous skeleton, with each joint having specific ligamentous attachments that support joint integrity and guide motion. Each joint is moved by muscular action that crosses single and multiple joints. The muscular elements are contained within fascial supporting structures. Primary dysfunction resulting in asymmetric motion of these structures causes tissue overload, inflammation, and secondary nociception. Manipulative treatment is directed toward restoring symmetric normal joint motion, muscle tone, ligamentous strength and length, and symmetry of tension within all myofascial elements.

Neurologic Model

The human nervous system is the most complex and sophisticated in the animal kingdom. Every body movement and function is governed and fine-tuned according to communication of stimuli from the internal and external environments. These can be broken down into three major reflex pathways to help us understand their function and how they inter-relate.

The somato-somatic reflex consists of afferent information from nociceptors, mechanoreceptors, and proprioceptors in the skin, muscle, joints, and tendons, synapsing on an anterior horn cell, which causes skeletal muscle to respond to external stimuli. These reflexes assist in orienting our bodies in space and performing the physical activities of daily living.

Visceral-visceral reflexes consist of afferent visceral sensory information synapsing in the intermediolateral cell column of the spinal cord and passing through the sympathetic lateral chain ganglion, or collateral ganglia, to synapse with the postganglionic motor fiber to the target organ. The target organs include the internal viscera as well as the skin viscera. Influence on pilomotor, vasomotor, and secretory motor activity of the skin results in palpable changes in the presence of somatic dysfunction.

Crossover from the somatic to visceral reflex arcs occurs in both directions. Visceral somatic reflexes account for lower right quadrant abdominal muscle spasm associated with appendicitis. Somatovisceral reflexes are less understood, but research evidence supports their presence and influences on visceral function.[25] Alteration of sympathetic nervous system (SNS) activity may compromise the body's immune system.[1, 27] Through SNS reflex responses, intervertebral movement may alter the discharge of adrenal and renal sympathetic nerve fibers,[24] and through these mechanisms that autonomic nervous system regulates visceral function in response to musculoskeletal demands.

It is through the neurobiochemistry of the neurotransmitters, endorphins, enkephalins, and substance P that biomechanical alteration of the musculoskeletal system affects the neuroendocrine axis. The trophic function of the nervous system maintains morphology and function by the antegrade and retrograde transport of complex protein and lipid substances along neurons and across synapses to the target organ.

Respiratory/Circulatory Model

The maintenance of cellular health depends on the supply of elements necessary for metabolism and appropriate removal of waste products. The musculoskeletal system can influence circulation by bony or myofascial tension or compression of arterial, venous, and lymphatic systems. The venous and lymphatic systems are low-pressure, thin-walled systems lacking the driving force of the heart, and they depend on the muscles of the extremities and the thoracoabdominal diaphragm for propulsion. The musculoskeletal system has extensive attachment to the diaphragm, including the upper lumbar vertebra, lower six ribs, xiphoid process of the sternum, and the myofascial connections of the psoas and quadratus lumborum muscles with the lower extremities. The diaphragm creates negative intrathoracic pressure and "milks" the inferior vena cava, assisting in venous and lymphatic return via the vena cava and cisterna chyli. Alterations of any of these elements of the musculoskeletal system, including the cervical spine through phrenic nerve innervation, can influence respiratory and circulatory function. Disruption of segmentally mediated SNS outflow can influence vasomotor tone and subsequent target organ blood flow.

MAJOR CONCEPTS

In addition to choosing a model for patient treatment, other concepts enter into decision making.

Holistic Concepts

Holistic medicine emphasizes the interrelation of the musculoskeletal system with the other body systems. Because disorders of the internal organs often manifest themselves in the musculoskeletal system, and vice versa, the total patient, and not just one element, needs to be evaluated for successful treatment to occur.

Energy-Expending Concept

The musculoskeletal system, which makes up more than 60% of the human organism, is the major expender of body energy. Musculoskeletal dysfunction resulting in decreased efficiency increases the demand for energy during normal or increased activity and can be detrimental to the person who already has a compromised cardiovascular or pulmonary system.

Self-Regulating Concept

There are literally thousands of self-regulatory mechanisms operating within the body at all times. These homeostatic mechanisms are essential for the maintenance of health and, if altered by disease or injury, need to be restored. The goal of the physician should be to enhance, and not to interfere with, the body's self-regulating mechanisms to assist in the recovery from disease. The more this is done without the potential detrimental side effects of foreign substances, the greater enhancement of the patient's ability to recover.

NEUROLOGY OF THE MUSCULOSKELETAL SYSTEM

The neurologic control of musculoskeletal function is highly complex, underemphasized, and poorly understood. A comprehensive understanding of the clinical relevance of intricate pathways and reflex mechanisms gives better diagnostic accuracy than do generalized "strains and sprains" descriptions.

Mechanoreceptors and Nociceptors

Four classes of mechanoreceptors and nociceptors have been extensively described by Wyke[30] and have various functions and distributions throughout the soft tissues and joints. Type I mechanoreceptors are found in superficial layers of joint capsules and ligaments, have a low threshold, adapt slowly, fire continuously under tension, and relay joint position. Depending on position and speed of motion, they provide tonic reflexogenic effects, especially in the neck, hip, and shoulder, for postural stability. Type II mechanoreceptors are low-threshold, dynamic, and fast-adapting and continuously reflect change in tension. They are found in the deep layers of the joint capsule-especially in the lumbar spine, feet, hands, and temporomandibular joint. Type III mechanoreceptors are high-threshold and very slow adapting and are found in the deep and superficial layers of joint ligaments of the extremities and superficial layers of joint capsules in the lumbar spine. Type IV nociceptors are nonadaptive, high-threshold receptors found in joint capsules, articular fat pads, anterior dura mater, spinal ligaments and connective tissue, and blood vessels, except in the brain. They are found in vessels associated with muscles and nerve but not directly in these structures. Mechanoreceptor stimulation by stretch, oscillation, or pressure can either inhibit or facilitate reflex activities or macroreceptors.

Golgi Tendon Receptors

Golgi tendon receptors are located in the musculotendinous junction in tendons and respond to tension via 1B afferent fibers traveling to the spinal cord. Tension produced by stretch or active contraction of muscle fibers in series with the golgi tendon apparatus reflexively inhibits motor neurons to their muscle of origin and stimulates more neurons of the antagonist. This reflex pathway balances excitatory input and protects against excessive muscle contraction. It appears that the therapeutic benefit of muscle energy techniques and of postcontraction muscle stretch[12] uses this reflex pathway.

Muscle Spindles

The muscle spindles have two types of intrafusal fibers arranged in parallel with the extrafusal muscle fibers, each with different sensory and motor innervation. Intrafusal fibers are innervated by thin axonal gamma motor neurons originated in the ventral horn. Sensation from the primary annulospiral and secondary flower-spray receptors carry afferent information via 1A and group-two axons to the cord and synapse with gamma efferents to form the "gamma loop." The primary endings respond to the velocity of stretch (joint motion) and length (joint position), with the secondary endings responding only to length. The spindle afferents, directly and through interneurons, influence alpha motor neuron activity to corresponding homonymous muscle and, through polyneuronal pathways, to its synergist. The spindle is sensitive to and reports the relative length of extrafusal fibers to intrafusal fibers. Extrafusal and intrafusal fiber disparity leads to increased muscle contraction to silence the spindle. As a muscle shortens in response to alpha motor neurons, gamma neurons inform the intrafusal fiber to take up the slack and keep the "gain" constant over changes in length. This reflex activity is influenced positively during sleep, when relaxation of the spindles occurs, and negatively with high anxiety, when spindle tension is high and slight tension activates afferents.

Sympathetic Nervous System in Musculoskeletal Function

The autonomic nervous system is responsible for the control of visceral function in response to muscular demand. The parasympathetic division and sympathetic division have quite different actions but work conjointly to control total body function. The parasympathetic division innervates the visceral organs and tissues through the cranial nerves and sacral segments of the spinal cord. The SNS influences all of the tissues of the body, including the nervous system itself. Divergent neuronal pathways prevail, with synapsing preganglionic axons to sympathetic chain ganglion to diffuse postganglionic axons reinforced by circulating epinephrine and norepinephrine to influence tissue function. SNS divergent and selective convergent activity assists its ergotropic function,[8] adjusting circulatory, metabolic, and visceral activity to musculoskeletal demand. Central activation of the entire sympathetic division occurs during exertion, emergency, or environmental extremes. Motor activity through somatic innervation from the spinal cord also requires coordinated activity of the SNS.[21] Constant somatoautomatic integration of motor neuron and sympathetic preganglionic neurons in the cord requires coordination at segmental levels, as well as modulation by descending pathways from higher centers.

Desired movement patterns and their peripheral end organs dictate recruitment of neurons, and subsequent sensory inputs are distributed in a multisegmental fashion. Segmentation is an evolutionary response to the bony column, and bunching of nerve fibers into compact spinal roots reflects anatomic location, not function. Segmental influence is therefore appreciated only in dysfunction and not in normal neurophysiology.[20]

Facilitated Segment

A facilitated segment is defined as "a spinal segment that is influenced selectively over its dorsal roots, resulting in local spinal cord neurons maintaining a hyperexcitable (lower reflex threshold) state to all afferent impulses, producing sensory, motor, and autonomic manifestations."[18] Impulses from the cutaneous receptors, postural and equilibrium centers, and the cerebral cortex all converge on spinal neurons. If this neuronal stimulus is sufficient, it maintains the spinal segment in a continuous state of excessive activity. Increases in peripheral stimulation from postural, mechanical, and articular dysfunction can elicit a response through central connections and through the SNS that is disproportional to the amount of afferent stimulation. This may create many symptoms, including alteration in peripheral tissue texture due to increased vasomotor activity and sweat gland secretor motor activity due to facilitated sympathetic nervous system reflexes.

Aberrant activity of the sympathetic nervous system affects peripheral receptors by lowering their thresholds, facilitating neuromuscular transmission[11] and facilitating the central nervous system's synaptic transmission, resulting in a central excitatory state.[17] The resultant increased nervous system activity leads to sympathetic sensory and motor changes mainfested as tender points,[19] myofascial trigger points,[29] and spondylogenic reflex syndromes.[26] The facilitated segment is a lesion on which irritation is focused from mechanoreceptors and other peripheral and central stimuli.[16]

The central nervous system affects motor activity in a "vertical alpha–gamma connection" by directing specific activity through the thalamus, basal ganglia, cerebellum, and cortex and by supporting postural activity from the brain stem, reticular formation, reticulospinal tracts, lateral vestibular center, and the rubrospinal tract.[10] Vegetative and emotional effects on gamma activity are influenced by the thalamocortical and pallidum systems via the brain stem.[10]

Central nervous system spindle sensitivity may be preset for anticipated movement patterns. Maladaption with high gamma spindle sensitivity occurs in tension and anxiety states and situations perceived to be threatening. Somatic dysfunction can occur when intrafusal and extrafusal fiber forces have not been centrally ordered.[19] Persistent disparity of gamma firing may well explain the palpable sense of "bind," as opposed by relative ease in normal tissues. The increased tissue tension felt in somatic dysfunction may be purely neuromuscular rather than of intra-articular nature.

One cannot discuss the neurology of the musculoskeletal system and the role of somatic dysfunction without addressing the issue of pain. A skilled manual medicine practitioner can identify somatic dysfunction in many asymptomatic patients. What then is the role of somatic dysfunction in musculoskeletal pain syndromes? Clinical experience has shown that significant somatic dysfunction with motion restriction may be a component part of the patient's presentation in areas that are not the primary pain site. Treatment appropriate to these dysfunctions has been shown to assist in relief of the painful area. In other instances, the somatic dysfunction itself may well be the pain generator in the area of primary pain complaint, and appropriate treatment resolves the pain presentation. Inhibition of pain occurs by three mechanisms: (1) Stimulation of mechanoreceptors by articulation reduces basal levels of substance P in the spinal cord, thereby reducing transmission of afferents from type IV receptors for as long as 4 to 6 minutes. (2) High-intensity afferent inhibitory stimulus from lower neurons to the reticular activating formulation from a high-velocity thrust generating fast stretch and low tension, vibrations of 100 to 140 Hz,[30] extreme temperatures of heat and cold, and intense emotions, i.e., sex, fear, and pain can last 6 to 8 months. (3) Inhibition by central nervous system descending pathways with release of endorphins and enkephalins stimulated by electroacupuncture of 4 Hz.[23a] Paradoxically, the area of major restriction in somatic dysfunction is not necessarily where the pain presentation is but is related to the relative hypermobility of the tissues related to the restricted segment. Acuteness and chronicity of the dysfunction also affect the pain presentation. Acute dysfunctions with muscle spasm and tissue inflammation present and respond differently than do chronic dysfunctions, which influences the choice of the type of manipulation to be used in the "manipulative prescription."

MANUAL MEDICINE ARMAMENTARIUM

Structural diagnosis and manual medicine techniques require that the practitioner have a comprehensive knowledge of the clinical anatomy of the region. The anatomy of the vertebral column demonstrates differences within the cervical, thoracic, and lumbar regions. The typical cervical (C3–7), thoracic, and lumbar vertebra all have vertebral bodies with intervening intervertebral discs and posterior arches, including the pedicles, lamina, articular processes, transverse processes, and spinous processes. In the cervical region the articular facets and processes support a considerable amount of weight, whereas in the thoracic and lumbar regions the weight is supported more on the vertebral bodies and intervertebral discs. The facet facings determine the amount and type of motion available. Flexion and extension are permitted in all regions, but the amount of sidebending and rotation varies greatly, being limited in the lumbar region and with considerable mobility within the cervical region. The intervertebral foramina are of major significance because they relate the dorsal and ventral roots forming the mixed nerve, which arises from the canal to innervate local and distant structures. Altered anatomy from a pathologic process such as spondylosis and spondylarthrosis can compromise the intervertebral canal. So, too, can dysfunction of the apophyseal joint. Both structural and dysfunctional alteration of the anatomy can occur singly but usually does so in combination. Because of the extensive mechanoreceptor and nociceptor innervation of the arthrodial joints, particularly in the cervical spine, alteration in joint function can reflexly influence both anterior and primary division of the spinal nerve. The arthrodial joint, posterior ligamentous structures of the vertebral motion segment, and related segmental paravertebral muscles are all innervated through the posterior primary division of the spinal nerve.

Articular hypertrophic changes, coupled with disc degeneration, can reduce the craniocaudal diameter of the intervertebral foramina. During the degenerative cascade[14] there is a phase of relative hypermobility when the arthrodial joints are more loose than normal. The cascade ends with hypomobility due to both bony and ligamentous hypertrophy. This is viewed as resulting in greater "stability" of the vertebral motion segment; however, for total vertebral column mobility to be maintained, vertebral motion segments not involved in the degenerative process attempt to compensate with relative hypermobility in adjacent segments. The challenge in structural diagnosis is appropriate diagnosis of hypomobility due to osseous pathology, hypomobility due to dysfunction, and relative hypermobility due to compensatory mechanisms.

Another process accompanying both anatomic pathologic and dysfunctional pathology of the vertebral axis is associated disturbance of muscle coordination. Altered muscle function can span the spectrum of proprioceptive sensory motor imbalance to altered muscle firing pattern sequence, with resultant tightness of some muscle groups and relative weakness of others. It is for this reason that appropriate exercise programming is such an essential component of patient care when manual medicine procedures are used.

MANUAL MEDICINE TECHNIQUES

Soft tissue manipulation mechanically and neuroreflexively improves the functional capacity of tight tissues, particularly in muscle hypertonicity and spasm. The treatment goal is to overcome muscle spasm, create symmetric motion, and reduce passive congestion, which always accompanies immobility. Examples of mechanical and reflexive soft tissue mechanisms include Chapman's reflexes, Travell's trigger points, acupressure, myofascial release, message, Trager, and Rolfing.

Articulatory manipulation includes mobilization with and without impulse. The goal is to obtain maximal symmetric articular range of motion and to stimulate mechanoreceptors creating either facilitory or inhibitory responses both centrally and peripherally. Mobilization without impulse includes a repetitive oscillatory operator force enhancing the overall range of motion. This can be graded from one to four in force level. Mobilization with impulse uses a rapidly accelerating, operator-induced force of short amplitude, frequently resulting in an associated joint "pop," or cavitation phenomenon, with the end point of improving articular mobility and the reduction of associated muscle hypertonicity.

Any of the soft tissue or articulatory procedures can be classified as direct or indirect methods, depending on whether the activating force is against the resistive barrier or in a direction directly opposite.

The activating force of manipulation can be classified as *extrinsic,* coming from outside the patient's body, and includes operator guiding, springing, or thrusting and assisting forces such as gravity, straps, pads, or traction. Activating forces from within the body are classified as *intrinsic* and include respiration, muscle contraction, and the inherent nervous system reflexes to keep the body posturally oriented to its environment.

Most of the commonly used manipulation procedures act directly and use extrinsic activating forces, such as mobilization with and without impulse, and intrinsic activating forces of muscle contraction (muscle energy technique).

Indirect techniques depend more on the intrinsic neurologic reflex mechanisms and involve positioning the dysfunctional joint at its point of maximal ease away from both the normal and the restrictive barriers and maintaining that position for sufficient time to reduce afferent mechanoreceptor and nociceptor activity. Theoretically, the muscle is shortened to its point of "ease" until the disparity between intrafusal and extrafusal fiber firing is overcome and results in restoring the short, tight muscle to a more normal resting length. Examples of indirect techniques include Jones' strain/counterstrain, release by position, "balance and hold technique," and dynamic functional technique.

When one understands the biomechanics and the neurology of the system, a wide variety of techniques can be developed and used as appropriate for the patient presentation.

Once symmetrical motion has been restored, it is necessary to coordinate neuromuscular balance through patient-directed positional and balance training and therapeutic exercise. Hypermobile areas are stabilized through segmental exercise of deep rotary and multifidi muscles. Increased endurance and strength of muscle occur through exercise to help maintain the gains established by manipulation and to restore maximal pain-free movement in postural balance.

FACTORS INFLUENCING MANIPULATIVE CARE

Factors influencing manipulative care include patient age and general physical condition, acuteness or chronicity of the problem, operator size and ability, equipment available, and effectiveness of previous and present therapy.

Advanced age is associated with conditions such as spondylosis, spondylarthrosis, and osteoporosis, which may argue against mobilization with impulse technique but still are amenable to the less traumatic soft-tissue and indirect procedures.

The general condition of the patient determines the capacity to undergo manipulation. A compromised cardiac or respiratory state would rule against the use of a prolonged isometric contraction as part of muscle energy technique and would reduce the length of treatment time at each intervention.

Manual medicine procedures need to be prescribed as precisely as any other therapeutic modality. The practitioner needs to determine which type is most appropriate, how much per intervention, how frequently, and for what period. Manipulative treatment is designed to maximize the functional capacity of the musculoskeletal system and must deal with the anatomy as presented. Altered anatomy can occur because of developmental variations, trauma, and previous surgery. The manual medicine procedure would be modified, depending on these factors. Precision of treatment is essential so that hypermobility is prevented in normal segments and the hypomobility of dysfunctional segments is overcome.

Alteration in the anatomy, such as degenerative disc disease with bulging and even herniation, would modify the manipulative prescription. Herniated intervertebral discs are not necessarily an absolute contraindication for manipulation but require high levels of diagnostic and therapeutic skill.

Manipulative care appears to have a broader impact than just altering the biomechanics of the anatomy. There are complex neurochemical, neuroendocrine, and psychological outcomes as well. A hands-on therapeutic approach by a health practitioner appears to have a positive impact on levels of wellness of a patient. Whether this is neurochemical, psychological, or a combination of both is unknown at this time, but the observation is most common. After manipulative treatment the patient frequently experiences a sense of enhanced well-being, similar to the euphoric high following administration of some pharmaceutical substance. Frequently, this sense of well-being lasts only a short period, and the patient returns on a frequent basis for additional manipulative treatment to obtain this high. Both the patient and the physician must be aware of the potential for addictive behavior in the use of manipulative treatment.

Manipulation should be given frequently and over sufficient time to obtain maximal functional capacity of the musculoskeletal system. This may be achieved before full pain relief occurs. In prescribing manipulative treatment, the following principles apply. In acute conditions, the patient is seen more frequently, with less intense manipulation at each visit. In chronic conditions, the patient is seen less frequently but is manipulated more intensively at each visit. In chronic recurrent conditions in which the altered functional anatomy cannot ever be restored to normal, a structured 2- to 3-month visit schedule is frequently sufficient to maintain the patient's functional capacity at maximum.

CONTRAINDICATIONS

Contraindications are classsified as absolute and relative. Perhaps the only absolute contraindication is high-velocity thrust with hypermobility. Otherwise, contraindications are dependent on accurate diagnosis and use of an appropriate procedure. Relative contraindications include primary bone and joint disease, metabolic bone disease, primary or secondary malignant bone disease, genetic disorders (e.g., Down syndrome), and progressive neurologic deficits, including radiculopathy and long tract cord signs. Caution in the manipulation of the cervical spine is always appropriate, because of the vulnerability of the vertebral artery. Hyperextension and rotation are to be avoided both diagnostically and therapeutically.

Accurate and adequate diagnostic procedures and the choice of an appropriate manual medicine treatment plan can avoid complications.

INCIDENCE OF COMPLICATIONS

Fortunately, the complication rate of manual medicine is low, ranging between 1 in 400,000[3] to 1 in 1,000,000.[7] A distinction is made between symptom exacerbation, which occurs in approximately 1 in 40,000[3] and a true complication by pathologic change. Symptom exacerbation can be anticipated in many patients, particularly those with long-standing biomechanical and reflex changes in the musculoskeletal system. Complications should be avoided, because the outcome of many is frequently disastrous, particularly those involving the central nervous system through compromise of the vertebral basilar artery system.[5]

PAIN SYNDROMES AND MANIPULATIVE MEDICINE
MODELS—CLINICAL EXAMPLES

Having established a basis for the rationale for structural diagnosis and manual medicine treatment—when and why to treat somatic dysfunction—we portray its use through common clinical syndromes seen in office practice. Because of the complexity of multiple factors, musculoskeletal pain syndromes are innately variable among patients. This demands evaluation of the whole musculoskeletal system, avoiding tunnel vision regarding the particular region of symptomatology.

Failed Low Back Syndrome—Postural Structural Model

The postural/structural model emphasizes the osseous skeleton and its symmetry of motion and is useful in evaluating the failed low back syndrome. Structural evaluation of the gait demonstrates the small amount of innominate rotation around the sacrum, with the symphysis pubis rotating about a transverse axis. The entire pelvis rotates around a vertical axis, and the lumbomechanics of lumbar spine show sidebending and rotation as coupled motions to opposite sides.[5]

Dysfunctions of the lumbar spine and pelvis altering the biomechanics of the normal gait are commonly seen in the failed low back syndrome. "The dirty half dozen" are six dysfunctions seen in 95% of patients with failed low back pain.[6]

The first is pubic dysfunction. Normally, the pelvis moves around the pubis during walking, and the pube is the most stable part of the pelvis. A superior-inferior shear maneuver, which restricts the normal rotary mobility of the pubis, interferes with all other elements of normal gait.

The second is nonadaptive lumbar spine mechanics, with restriction of sidebending and rotation to the same side, most commonly associated with restriction of extension. This motion restriction accompanies the clinical presentation of "the posterior facet syndrome" and frequently responds to appropriate manual medicine treatment.

The third is the anatomic short-leg, pelvic-tilt syndrome with compensatory lumbar scoliosis. Discrepancy of 1/4 inch is identified in 20% to 30% of the asymptomatic population, with 55% to 70% of the symptomatic population having discrepancy of 6 mm, and 90% with 12 mm being symptomatic.[28] The body attempts to compensate for this discrepancy by rotating one innominate anteriorly to lengthen the short leg or posteriorly to shorten the long leg. The lumbar spine assumes an ipsilateral convexity and restricts mobility of sidebending to, and rotation away, from the short-leg side. Manipulative treatment is directed toward correction of lumbar mechanics, innominate rotations, and the appropriate use of lift therapy to bring the pelvis to balance.

The fourth is innominate shear dysfunction, a nonphysiologic motion of the innominate in a superior or inferior "slip" upon the sacrum. This occurs in patients who are anatomically disposed by a more parallel joint surface at the sacroiliac joint with loss of joint beveling and the convex concave relationship. The trauma of a fall on the buttock or other superior loading of a lower extremity can result in a superior innominate shear (upslip), and a long-axis traction injury, such as a forward motion of the trunk with fixation of the lower extremity, can result in an inferior shear (downslip). Both are associated with pain in the lower back, buttock, and posterior thigh. The extent of disability is greater than anticipated by type of injury reported.

The fifth is lack of normal anterior nutation of the sacrum, a motion required for extension of the trunk. Backward sacral torsions or extended sacra restrict anterior nutation of the sacral base. They are frequently associated with nonadaptive lumbar mechanics, particularly extension restriction with loss of the normal lumbar lordosis. Patients with this condition mimic radiculopathy associated with disc disease and frequently have some sensory changes, occasional weakness, and mildly diminished deep tendon reflexes but lack hard electromyographic changes. This condition is frequently found in patients who have not been responsive to surgical intervention.

The sixth dysfunction is alteration in muscle balance of the lower extremities and trunk. Asymmetric lower extremity and trunk muscle function results in biomechanical asymmetry of the pelvis and lower back. Of particular importance is the balance of the hip flexors, the iliopsoas and rectus femoris, and the functional capacity of the erector spinae. Tightness of the piriformis is frequently seen asymmetrically and alters normal rotational motion of the hip. This muscle not only interferes with biomechanical function but also can entrap the sciatic nerve, resulting in radiating thigh and leg pain simulating a classic radiculopathy (the piriformis syndrome).[28] Jull and Janda[12] have described abnormal muscle firing patterns with tight strong iliopsoas and upper erector spinae muscles reflexively inhibiting the abdominals and gluteus maximus ("crosspelvic pattern"), which results in inability to stabilize the pelvis. These altered muscle firing patterns can be retrained with appropriate sensory motor balance training followed by stretching and then restrengthening. Any exercise program prescribed for patients with failed low back pain, including machine-assisted, must take this altered firing pattern phenomena in consideration.

Wrist Pain: A Structural Model

In evaluating a patient for wrist pain, all nonstructural diagnoses must be ruled out. These include radicular pain, reflex sympathetic dystrophy, carpal tunnel syndrome, deQuervain's syndrome, tenosynovitis, trigger fingers, and degenerative and inflammatory arthritis. Wrist pain may still be present in the absence of all of the above. The wrist is not a single joint but a region comprising multiple joints. The motions within the carpal bones, of the carpal bones in relation to the radius and ulna, and with the metacarpals are governed by their relative convexities, concavities, and translatory movements. Each of these joints has an element of joint play,[23] and the involuntary joint play movements must be present for normal pain-free voluntary motion at the wrist. The details of all of these joint motions are beyond the scope of this presentation, but a few of the more common ones resulting in painful restriction are presented. Limited wrist extension is commonly associated with restriction of the capitate moving on the lunate. Restriction of the scaphoid and lunate on the distal radius is frequently associated in restriction of wrist flexion. Proper mobilization of these and other joint play movements within the wrist restores normal, pain-free movement at the wrist region. Altered joint play at the wrist frequently accompanies the classic carpal tunnel syndrome. Frequently, restoration of joint play, along with other nonoperative measures, is sufficient to prevent the need for surgical treatment of this condition.

Cervical Spine and Related Pain Syndromes

The cervical spine is frequently involved in a number of pain syndromes including the cervical syndrome (pain in the neck), the cervical cranial syndrome (pain in the neck plus headache), and the cervical brachial syndrome (pain in the neck with radiation to the upper extremity). The cervical spine is influenced by alteration and function of almost every other element in the musculoskeletal system. Head position and its relation to the upper extremities and thoracic spine can be altered by dysfunction anywhere within the body, including the pelvic girdle. Muscular balance of the neck and upper extremity is frequently altered with strong pectoralis major and minor muscles anteriorly and the upper trapezius posteriorly.[12] The resulting protracted scapula, humerus, and clavicle and internally rotated humerus create forces on the cervical spine that lead to the classic forward head posture. This can negatively influence the neurophysiology of the cervical and brachial plexus. Dysfunction in the upper cervical spine is frequently related to headache, dizziness, and visual disturbances and appears to relate to the innervation through the cervical plexus. The sympathetic nervous system control of the vasomotor tone of the intracranial structures is also apparently influenced by dysfunction in the upper cervical vertebral complex. Involvement of the lower cervical segments can contribute to many shoulder and arm syndromes. Excellent correlation between clinically observed facet dysfunction and provocative facet injection has been shown.[13, 22]

Headaches related to cervical dysfunction are of several types. Gutmann[7] describes a "hypomobility headache" due to "joint locking," most frequently of the upper cervical spine but also of the mid-to-lower cervical spine, upper ribs, and upper thoracic spine. Hypermobility headaches are constant in nature and occur in prolonged postures with the head in end range. Static headache, or postural headache, occurs with insufficient biomechanical compensation for static problems, such as scoliosis due to pelvic obliquity or leg length discrepancy and associated abnormal muscle compensation, creating tension in the suboccipital muscles.

Dizziness is a frequent symptom accompanying neck pain, headaches, and temporomandibular joint dysfunction. Dizziness can result from disturbed sensory information from the labyrinth, optical organs, and proprioceptive system. The mechanoreceptors of the upper cervical spine contribute greatly to the orientation of the body to three-dimensional space. Altered function of this region can contribute to a sensation of dizziness.

The manual medicine practitioner working with the cervical spine must be aware of the relation of the vertebral artery. Because of the anatomic relation of the vertebral artery to the cervical spine, marked extension and rotation of the head on the neck can compromise the normal vertebral artery, leading to basilar insufficiency. If vascular disease of the vertebral and carotid systems occurs concurrently, the practitioner must be careful about manipulative intervention to the cervical spine. Cervical-related dizziness treated with soft-tissue and articulatory manipulation in a limited population study showed good-to-excellent responses to treatment.[10]

The cervical brachialgias, particularly those related to the thoracic outlet syndrome, require a comprehensive evaluation of the cervical spine, thoracic spine, upper rib cage, and clavicle. Somatic dysfunction in these areas can influence the brachial plexus and its branches, both reflexively and by combined compression and inflammation. Cervical mechanics affect scalene function, which can elevate the first and second ribs. Muscle imbalance between the pectoralis minor and the posterior scapular stabilizers can compress the neurovascular bundle. Restoration of maximal function to the cervical spine, rib cage, and clavicle can result in reduction of pain complaints throughout the upper extremity, including those frequently related to the shoulder (bursitis), the elbow (epicondylitis), and the wrist (carpal tunnel syndrome).

CONCLUSION

Musculoskeletal pain syndromes present a serious challenge to the health care delivery system, particularly to practitioners of physical medicine and rehabilitation. A working knowledge of the role of structural diagnosis and manual medicine techniques can be of assistance to the practitioner who understands the principles of their application. As in any other diagnostic or therapeutic tool, study and practice are necessary for the achievement of competency.

References

1. Besedovsky H, Delrey A, Sorkin E, et al: Immunoregulation mediated by the sympathetic nervous system. Cell Immunol 48:346–355, 1979
2. Dorland's Illustrated Medical Dictionary, ed 25. Philadelphia, WB Saunders, 1981
3. Dvorak J, Orelli F: How dangerous is manipulation to the cervical spine? Manual Medicine 2:1–4, 1985
4. Greenman PE: Principles of Manual Medicine. Baltimore, Williams & Wilkins, 1989
5. Greenman PE: Clinical aspects of sacroiliac function in walking. Journal of Manual Medicine 5:125–130, 1990
6. Greenman PE: Sacroiliac dysfunction in the failed low back pain syndrome. In Proceedings, First Interdisciplinary Congress on Low Back Pain and Its Relation to the Sacroiliac Joint, San Diego, CA, 1992
7. Gutmann G: Injuries to the verterbral artery caused by manual therapy. Manuelle Medizin 21:2–14, 1983
8. Hess WR: The Diencephalon—Autonomic and Extrapyramidal Functions. New York, Grune and Stratton, 1954
9. Holt S, Yates PO: Cervical spondylosis and nerve root lesions. J Bone Joint Surg [Br] 48:407, 1966
10. Hotvedt P: Dizziness related to cervical pathology. Scientific Physical Therapy 1:1990
11. Hutter OF, Loewenstein WR: Nature of neuromuscular facilitation by sympathetic stimulation in the frog. J Physiol [Lond] 130:559–571, 1955
12. Jull GA, Janda V: Muscles and motor control in low back pain: Assessment and management. In Twomey LT, Taylor JR (eds): Physical Therapy of the Low Back. New York, Churchill Livingstone, 1987
13. Jull G, Bogduk N, Marsland A: The accuracy of manual diagnosis for cervical zygatophysial joint pain syndromes. Med J Aust 148:233–237, 1988
14. Kirkaldy-Willis WH: The pathology and pathogenesis of low back pain. In Kirkaldy-Willis WH (ed): Managing Low Back Pain. New York, Churchill Livingstone, 1983
15. Kleynhans AM: Complications of and contraindications to spinal manipulative therapy. In Haldeman S (ed): Modern Developments in the Principles and Practice of Chiropractic. New York, Appleton Century Crofts, 1980
16. Korr IM: The neural basis of the osteopathic lesion. J Am Osteopath Assoc 47:191–198, 1947
17. Korr IM: The sympathetic nervous system as mediator between the somatic and supportive processes. In The Physiologic Basis of Osteopathic Medicine. 1970, pp 21–38
18. Korr IM: The facilitated segment: A factor in injury to body framework. In The Collected Papers of Irwin Korr. Newark, OH, American Academy of Osteopathy, 1973
19. Korr IM: Proprioceptors and somatic dysfunction. In The Collected Papers of Irwin Korr. Newark, OH, American Academy of Osteopathy, 1975
20. Korr IM: The spinal cord as organizer of disease processes: Some preliminary perspectives. J Am Osteopath Assoc 76:35–45, 1976
21. Korr IM: The spinal cord as organism of disease process: The peripheral autonomic nervous system. J Am Osteopath Assoc 79:82–90, 1979
22. Bogduk N: Cervical cause of headache and dizziness. In Grieve GP (ed): Modern Manual Therapy of the Vertebral column. New York, Churchill Livingstone, 1986
23. Mennell JM: Joint Pain: Diagnosis and Treatment Using Manipulative Techniques. Boston, Little, Brown, 1964
23a. Pomeranz B: The brain's opiates at work in acupuncture. New Scientist, January 6, 1977, pp 12–13
24. Sato A, Swenson R: Sympathetic nervous system response to mechanical stress of the spinal column in rats. J Manipulative Physiol Ther 7:141–147, 1984
25. Sato A, Schaible H, Schmidt R: Types of afferents from the knee joint evoking sympathetic reflexes in cat inferior cardia nerves. Neurosci Lett 39:71–75, 1983
26. Skjelbred I: Epicondylitis and Its Relationship to the Cervical Spine. Scientific Physical Therapy, March 1990

27. Stein-Werblowsky R: The sympathetic nervous system and cancer. Exp Neuro 42:97–100, 1974
28. Steiner C, Staubs C, Ganon M, et al: Piriformis syndrome: Pathogenesis, diagnosis and treatment. J Am Osteopath Assoc 87:318–323, 1987
29. Travell J, Simmons D: Myofascial Pain and Dysfunction—The Trigger Point Manual. Baltimore, Williams & Wilkins, 1983
30. Wyke BD: The neurology of joints. Ann R Coll Surg Eng 41:25–49, 1967

Address reprint requests to

Jonathan L. Ritson, MD
4801 N. Mullen
Tacoma, WA 98407

CHRONIC PAIN FOLLOWING HEAD INJURY

Michael T. Andary, MD, Frederick Vincent, MD,
and Peter C. Esselman, MD

In recent years, there have been an increasing number of reports that describe some of the problems arising in patients with traumatic brain injury (TBI) and coexistent chronic pain.[3, 54, 56] Although the literature does not give clear guidance on the incidence, etiology, or treatment of this problem, clinicians involved in the treatment of these patients are beginning to identify them as a subgroup of patients who require special consideration.[42] There is a large overlap of behaviors, signs, and symptoms in patients with the dual diagnosis of mild traumatic pain injury (MTBI) and chronic pain syndrome, including pain behaviors, memory and concentration problems, fatigue, impaired vocational performance, multiple medical contacts, dizziness, sleep disturbance, impaired social relationships, legal problems, myofascial tender points, anxiety, and depression.[3, 42, 57]

Identification of these patients is variable and at times difficult. Patients referred for chronic pain treatment may, on detailed evaluation, have a history of and sequelae of TBI. Among patients referred for chronic pain treatment, Anderson et al[3] described 11% (7/67) who had evidence for previously undiagnosed TBI. They used clinical criteria of cognitive changes and evidence of problems on their expanded mental status examination. Neuropsychological testing confirmed abnormalities in all five patients tested. The two other patients were not able to complete neuropsychological testing, because of funding problems for one and the refusal of testing in the other. These findings have not been replicated in any other study to date.

Approaching this problem from another angle, Uomoto and colleagues[54] systematically evaluated patients with identified TBI for complaints of chronic pain. Ninety-five per cent of those with mild TBI complained of a pain problem that interfered with daily activities, compared with only 22% of patients with moderate or severe TBI with this complaint. Headache was the most common

From Michigan State University, East Lansing, Michigan (MTA, FV); and University of
   Washington, Seattle, Washington (PCE)

PHYSICAL MEDICINE AND REHABILITATION CLINICS
OF NORTH AMERICA

VOLUME 4 • NUMBER 1 • FEBRUARY 1993

pain complaint and was seen in 89% of the mild TBI group and 18% of the moderate-to-severe group.

The literature is full of reports that discuss the postconcussive syndrome. As is often the case in medicine, the more names a problem has, the less the problem is understood. Other names for postconcussive syndrome include *minor contusion syndrome, posttraumatic vasomotor neurosis, posttraumatic nervous instability, posttraumatic syndrome, posttraumatic neurosis, railway spine, whiplash, minor traumatic brain injury,* and *mild head injury.*[1] The specific cause of these problems has not been clearly defined. Some sources have suggested that litigation and compensation are the primary motivators for these symptoms,[1, 41] but these assumptions are based on little more than anecdotal reports.

Because there are limited studies specifically addressing the dual diagnosis of MTBI and chronic pain, it would be helpful to explore the incidence of problems after MTBI and to review some of the prospective studies that have attempted to document these problems. It is very difficult to find out what happens to people who have MTBI, for numerous logistic and methodologic reasons; however, there have been some studies that can give us an idea of the relative incidence of symptoms and what kind of symptoms are involved. Rimel et al,[48] identified 535 hospital admissions for MTBI defined as loss of consciousness (LOC) of <20 minutes, admission Glasgow Coma Scale of ≥13, and less than 48 hours of hospital admission. Incredibly, they were able to get 3-month follow-up data on 424 of these patients. Of these, 79% continued to complain of headache, 59% had memory difficulties, and 14% were having difficulties with their activities of daily living. Most importantly, 34% of those employed at the time of injury were unemployed at 3-month follow-up. They were able to perform neuropsychological testing (Halstead-Reitan) on 69 of these patients, and overall, there was evidence for cognitive impairment on this testing. Only 6 of these 424 patients had initiated any litigation.

Another prospective and ambitious multicenter study attempted to address problems in methodology identified in a study by Rimel et al by identifying an appropriate socioeconomic control group and excluding subjects who had a history of TBI, a previous neuropsychological disorder, or ethanol or drug abuse. They measured neurobehavioral performance on neuropsychological tests and asked open-ended questions about postconcussive symptoms at 1 week, 1 month, and 3 months after MTBI. Their conclusion was that "single uncomplicated minor head injury *rarely* produces chronic *disability* or permanent cognitive impairment [emphasis added]." Close analysis of their results does not seem to support their conclusions for several reasons:

1. At the 3-month follow-up, the sample size was 32 patients of 155 identified. This shows a high rate of attrition and at 3 months, to use these researchers' words, "has little power to detect small gains" and small differences.
2. Incidence of postconcussion symptoms in these 32 patients was still very high at 3 months (47% had headache, 22% had decreased energy level, and 22% had dizziness).
3. There was no measure of what most rehabilitation specialists would consider disability (e.g., in employment, function, earning capacity, or activities of daily living).
4. If one is to assume that all of the patients lost to follow-up in their study had no symptoms (even though this is highly unlikely), at least 9% (14/155) would have symptoms. This can hardly be called rare.

When taken in context, their overall findings are very consistent with the incidence of problems following MTBI identified in other studies, and their data support the fact that there are continued pain complaints (at least headaches) in addition to other problems.

Dickmen and colleagues[12] prospectively followed up 20 MTBI patients and identified 20 controls who were friends of the patients and matched for age, sex, and education. Those studied were followed up at 1 month and 1 year with several measures, including symptoms, neuropsychological tests, and psychosocial measures, including the Sickness Impact Profile. At 1 month, they found that more than 50% of MTBI patients endured headaches, but less than 40% of controls did so; however, this difference was not statistically significant. At 1 year, there were minimal differences between the two groups, although there was a difference in the Sickness Impact Profile, with poorer function in alertness behavior and communication noted in the MTBI group. Pain complaints other than headache were not specifically reported.

Litigation, compensation, malingering, and other nonorganic issues have been cited as contributing to problems and even, by some, as the primary cause of the symptoms.[41] Several authors have attempted to eliminate litigation, compensation issues, or malingering as factors in their prospective studies. In New Zealand, a sample limited to young working men (thus limiting compensation factors and theoretically many of the more disabled people) who sustained MTBI, 20% (13/66) displayed symptoms at 90 days post injury, and 50% of those who could be found for follow-up (4/8) had symptoms that persisted after 2 years. There was no litigation in any of these cases, and all of these men had full return to work with diminished capacity despite these symptoms.[55] In Ireland, 14.5% (19/131) of patients continued to have symptoms after 1 year. They found that patients who were undergoing litigation had more symptoms than those who did not. Interestingly, they attempted to identify malingerers 6 weeks post injury and labeled 11% (15/131) as malingerers. On 1 year's follow-up, 9 of these 15 had no symptoms. The authors suggested that their highly subjective judgment of malingering was erroneous, and they did find symptoms in patients who were neither malingering nor in litigation, concluding that there are both organic and psychological causes for symptoms after MTBI.[49] A recent survey suggests that most clinicians think that compensation and litigation have some effect on postconcussion syndrome[37]; however, determining their role on patients' complaints continues to be difficult.[6]

When the prospective studies of MTBI are analyzed, the data strongly suggest that a significant portion of patients continue to have problems after MTBI even though they do not have litigation pending nor evidence for malingering. Although pain complaints have not been systematically documented, headache appears to be the most common problem. This strongly suggests that there are real problems that are associated with MTBI.

PHYSIOLOGICAL MECHANISMS

There are many more questions about this syndrome that are left unanswered. What are the anatomic, physiologic, and psychological mechanisms that contribute to the symptoms and behaviors that are seen after MTBI? Are the pain complaints from a central nervous system (CNS) injury, musculoskeletal or peripheral nerve injuries, behavioral or psychological factors, other unknown factors, or a combination of all the above? There appears to be evidence to suggest all of the above.

There are other complaints and unusual symptoms that patients with MTBI or the brain-pain syndrome present with and that warrant brief discussion here. Memory impairment, loss of awareness of the environment, atypical behaviors, déjà vu, and olfactory or visual auras (or both) may occur as ictal manifestations of temporal lobe epilepsy. Interictal behaviors such as hypergraphia, hypersexuality, and hyperreligiosity may also occur. Patients who exhibit symptoms consistent with temporal lobe seizures should be thoroughly evaluated with sleep electroencephalography (EEG) and (occasionally) 24-hour ambulatory EEG monitoring.

Dizziness and balance problems also are common after MTBI. Several possible causes include abnormalities in positional proprioceptors in the cervical and lumbar regions,[8, 24, 46] increased tone in cervical and lumbar regions, cervical sympathetic nerve abnormalities,[25] trigger points,[57] vestibular abnormalities,[57] and CNS damage.[34, 35] (See Zasler[57] for a more detailed discussion.)

Possible peripheral origins for pain after whiplash injuries include tears in muscles and ligaments,[38, 43a] greater occipital nerve neuralgia, nerve root irritation at the foramina,[57] myofascial dysfunction,[52] somatic dysfunction, cranial bone and cervical spine abnormalities,[29, 54a] migraine vascular spasm,[22] skull fractures and dural tears,[57] and cluster headache.[47]

The cause of the chronic pain may also be a CNS abnormality. There are many reports of CNS lesions that cause persistent or chronic pain complaints. Animal studies have shown that peripheral nociceptive input can cause physiologic plastic CNS changes that correlate with hyperalgesia or chronic painful states.[10, 14] Many pain researchers and clinicians believe that chronic pain states can be explained by CNS processing abnormalities and are not necessarily or primarily psychological.[19, 50] This finding is very hard to document in humans, but Andy[4] presents a case of chronic pain caused by brainstem seizures in a head injury patient, documented during implantation of a brain stimulation electrode.

Memory problems with cognitive difficulties have been associated with diffuse and focal structural and physiological CNS abnormalities.[23] Anatomic and physiologic CNS damage in humans with MTBI can often be hard or impossible to document, but newer techniques have been successful at documenting CNS dysfunction.[57] There are convincing studies showing physiologic abnormalities in animals subjected to MTBI.[27, 44, 45] There is evidence for neuropsychological abnormalities consistent with brain dysfunction and damage in MTBI, and whether or not the patient had LOC or litigation pending did not seem to matter.[5, 36, 48, 56] Further research on newer techniques to detect CNS injury is needed.

Memory problems, fatigue, and inadequate sleep are all symptoms common to people with MTBI, depression, headaches, anxiety and chronic pain. It is unclear what the physiologic mechanisms for the depression, anxiety, and other psychological manifestations are. Possibilities include primary brain injury causing mood changes, existing problems, psychological reaction to altered function or environment,[2, 17, 30] and a combination of factors. In most cases, it is probably impossible to sort out with confidence a specific cause for each symptom, and most cases are multifactorial. It becomes more difficult to determine from the literature the relation between pain, pain behavior, and CNS damage. There are numerous reports linking pain behavior to psychological, environmental, and thus CNS function.[18] If one considers that all observable behaviors stem from a series of biochemical reactions in the brain, it is hard to imagine that diffuse albeit mild brain injury will *not* significantly affect behavior. Theoretically, a patient with mild cognitive deficits that interfere with information processing and psychological function has impaired coping strategies and as a result may manifest excessive pain behaviors; however, there is limited evidence to support or refute this theory. Within the pain literature there is growing consensus and evidence that coping strategies are important in effectively functioning with chronic pain.[28] Although they do not necessarily reduce pain sensations, these coping techniques do control pain behaviors. One report showed that a significant proportion of outpatients in a clinic being seen for pain complaints have evidence for impaired cognition when they were systematically evaluated.[32] This finding suggests there may be cognitive and brain dysfunction problems in many of chronic pain patients, which could be a major contributor to their disability. The overlap and complex relation between brain function, psychology, pain, and behaviors are still poorly understood and extremely variable from person to person.

The incidence of low back pain after MTBI is unknown and has not been systematically studied. Braaf and Rosner[9] report low back pain in 42% of people with neck injuries in a retrospective review. As previously mentioned, Uomoto et al[54] have shown that 45% of patients with MTBI and seeking medical care report low back pain. It is not entirely clear whether this finding is due to associated injury to the low back, to the TBI, or to other causes and how it would compare with a control group.

At this stage of medical knowledge, it is safe to say that it is unknown why some people with chronic low back pain develop a chronic pain syndrome and become disabled whereas others are seemingly able to function despite their chronic pain. It is possible that part of the chronic pain syndrome may be due to impaired cognitive function or other CNS dysfunction.

DIAGNOSIS

The diagnosis of patients with the dual diagnosis necessitates recognizing and diagnosing both chronic pain and MTBI. Although there continues to be disagreement about the definition of chronic pain, it can be diagnosed in patients who have a pain "a month beyond . . . a reasonable time to heal" or at least 6 months after an injury.[7] Other factors that are associated include disability due to pain behaviors, impaired coping skills, no clear objective evidence for nociception, evidence of suffering, depressive symptoms, and other characteristics previously listed in this article.

MTBI can be more difficult to diagnose than chronic pain, because many people are willing to discuss somatic pain symptoms and less willing to admit to brain dysfunction. Additionally, cognitive deficits are harder to detect and document than are pain behaviors. Obtaining a history that suggests evidence for trauma significant enough to cause cognitive deficits is important. Unfortunately, there does not seem to be clear agreement on exactly how much trauma it takes to cause MTBI; some people with seemingly trivial impact have problems, whereas others with LOC and more severe injuries do not have any problems. LOC at the scene of the accident does not seem to be necessary to produce cognitive deficits.[36] There is also mounting evidence that cumulative, seemingly insignificant insults, such as heading a soccer ball or boxing, can cause brain dysfunction as measured by neuropsychological testing, EEG changes, and CT scan abnormalities.[21, 51, 53] Some authors have asked about both LOC or disorientation and whether the patient was "dazed" or not.[3, 36, 57] Other historical questions are necessary to delineate the patient's symptoms clearly and determine whether they are consistent with those seen in MTBI. Sorting through the history can be very difficult. On the one hand, patients may have agnosias or denial of deficits that make identification of problems difficult, and on the other hand, patients who are somatically focused may report many symptoms that are not medically relevant or helpful. Memory problems, impaired concentration, speech difficulties, perseveration, poor attention span, and other emotional and psychological symptoms are strongly suggestive of MTBI.

A traditional neurologic and physical examination focusing on and noting pain behaviors, range of motion, strength, myofascial tender points, gross neurologic deficits, and balance problems often is normal or consistent with a chronic pain syndrome. Anderson et al[3] suggest an additional mental status examination focusing on digit repetition and vigilance testing; new learning ability, demonstrating recall of a verbal story and four unrelated words; constructional testing, with reproduction of drawings; and proverb interpretation and similarities. They found these areas to be more helpful than other portions of the mental status examination.

There is no single test or series of tests that can clearly diagnose MTBI. Magnetic resonance imaging, CT scans, EEGs, and other tests are routinely normal or show nonspecific findings in any single patient with MTBI. Newer techniques such as single-photon emission CT, positron emission tomography, power spectral EEG analysis, brain electrical activity mapping, balance posturography, electronystagmography, electrooculography, autonomic nervous system evaluation, polysomnography, evoked potentials, and cognitive evoked potentials all show some promise in detecting mild brain dysfunction.[57] Unfortunately, these tests have been incompletely studied and are not widely available.

Neuropsychological testing is probably the most reliable available testing to assess for mild brain dysfunction. This testing should be done by an experienced neuropsychologist and needs to be focused on higher-level cognitive and integrative function such as judgment, interpretation, new learning ability, reasoning and planning skills, complex attention, ability to do two tasks simultaneously, memory, fine motor coordination, sensory-motor function, visual spatial function, language and communication, mood, and personality. Some of the standard neuropsychometric tests were initially designed for identifying focal brain injuries and are in the normal range for many patients with diffuse mild subcortical injury. Premorbid cognitive function must also be considered; for example, someone with a high premorbid intelligence and a college education may still score in the normal range on standardized testing despite what would be measured as a significant drop in performance. Cognitive perceptual motor testing, such as Southern California Integrative Testing, measures somatosensory integrative function, which is not routinely done in neuropsychologic testing and may be more sensitive to detect higher level integrative brain dysfunction.[58]

The final diagnosis of MTBI must take into account the patient's complete situation, including history, physical examination, and test results, to determine the diagnosis and identify deficits and problems that can be treated.

TREATMENT

The literature gives very little specific guidance for treatment of the myriad problems that can occur in patients with MTBI and chronic pain syndrome, and the fact that treatment is complicated suggests that approaches to these patients need to be established.[3, 54] Unfortunately, there have been limited studies detailing outcomes after treatment for TBI and chronic pain. In one brief report using a retrospective case control design, Andary et al[2a] compared treatment of dual diagnosis (MTBI and chronic pain syndrome) with that of chronic pain patients and found similar outcomes in full-time competitive employment (8/12 patients) in both groups. The dual-diagnosis group required longer treatment time (459 versus 294 days) than the chronic pain group.

Treatment is often geared toward the bias of each particular practitioner or clinic; thus, pain clinics treat the pain and pain behaviors, TBI clinics focus on brain injury issues, and individual professionals focus on their area of expertise (e.g., physical therapists on exercises, psychologists on psychotherapy, physicians on medications, chiropractors on manipulation, and so on). General recommendations have included early rehabilitation,[31] treatment in an operant pain program,[54] hypnotherapy,[40] or treatment using an eclectic and empiric approach.[42] Given the lack of programs for the dual diagnosis, it is worthwhile to consider treatments that have been used for either TBI or chronic pain. These treatments include medications, standard chronic pain treatment, psychotherapy, cognitive retraining, physical therapy, occupational therapy, speech pathology, nutritional counseling, vocational rehabilitation, recreational therapy, biofeedback, manual medicine, and various psychological counseling techniques. Any of the above combinations could theoretically be used in a multidisciplinary or interdisciplinary format in either an inpatient or outpatient setting.[26, 33, 42, 43, 54b, 57]

Treating the dual diagnosis as simple chronic pain has theoretic and practical problems that could interfere with treatment outcome. For example, using cognitive-behavioral strategies to deal with chronic pain may be difficult in patients who have impaired cognitive skills.[42] Conversely, addressing only cognitive problems may leave a patient with good cognitive skills but also with uncontrolled pain behaviors that make employment impossible.

Within our group of authors, there is not general agreement about the single best way to treat patients with TBI and chronic pain. One author (MA) prefers addressing the TBI issues first in an interdisciplinary team setting through a program of cognitive perceptual motor retraining[58]; improving physical performance (balance, strength, range of motion, and endurance); nutritional counseling; osteopathic manipulative therapy; and psychological counseling working on problem solving, social skills, coping techniques, stress management, family issues, and other deficit areas. All disciplines encourage independence in daily activities. Pain behaviors and passive modalities are discouraged during treatments. Other behaviors that impair function are identified. Consistent strategies to improve them are explained to the patient and reinforced by all members of the treatment team. Pain behaviors often become less of a problem when this approach is used. As patients improve, they undergo a prevocational evaluation, and if pain behaviors still interfere with function, the treatment focuses more on the specific pain behaviors, thus helping patients to improve their function and activity despite their pain. The focus of treatment then turns to vocational goals, and the vocational counselor becomes an integral part of the team. Formal therapy is gradually replaced with prevocational and vocational activities and supporting early employment effort when possible. Treatment, support, and follow-up are maintained, usually for the first few months of employment and then as needed.

Uomoto and Esselman[54] suggest that much of the disability from MTBI is due to problems with the chronic pain syndrome and that treatment of the pain behaviors in an interdisciplinary operant pain program can significantly improve function. When the chronic pain problem, and not cognitive dysfunction, is clearly the major factor limiting return to previous activities, the patient may best be treated in an operant pain program. This program should emphasize reactivating and improving physical functioning, educating the patient and family, decreasing pain behaviors, and psychological counseling.

Treating individual symptoms, e.g., headaches with nerve blocks or cognitive remediation, without addressing all the other problems the patient faces, e.g., vocational, family, and psychological issues, is likely to leave the patient with a less-than-satisfactory outcome. Some patients can be treated by the solo practitioner, but most of the complicated patients require multidisciplinary or more likely interdisciplinary treatment.

MEDICATIONS

Medications should be considered for treatment in these patients, and the general guidelines regarding the use of pain medications as outlined in the article by Buckley and Chabal in this issue should be used. Additionally, medications for headaches and seizures need to be considered in patients with TBI and chronic pain. Detailed review of this is beyond the scope of this article. Medications should be targeted for specific problems and specific symptoms, e.g., abortive medications (Midrin, Cafergot) for migraine headache, antidepressants for depression or headaches, and so on.[11, 15, 26]

EARLY INTERVENTION

Addressing problems early, as advocated throughout this issue and in the literature,[30, 31] is probably the most effective way to avoid problems in many patients. It remains to be proven whether systematic follow-up for all MTBI patients could prevent the disability, pain, and suffering that occur.

CONCLUSIONS

Patients with coexistent chronic pain and TBI are becoming recognized as a separate subgroup of patients with unique problems. The literature supports the fact that these problems regularly occur in a significant proportion of the population and are not due to malingering or compensation issues. Diagnosis of these problems, particularly the MTBI, is challenging, and there is no single test that confirms the diagnosis. Treatment issues are complicated and must take into account both diagnoses.

References

1. Adams RD, Victor M: Principles of Neurology. New York, McGraw-Hill, 1989
2. Alves WM: Natural history of post-concussive signs and symptoms. Physical Medicine & Rehabilitation: State of the Art Reviews 6:21–32, 1992
2a. Andary MT, Kulkarni MR, Haines C, et al: Traumatic brain injury/chronic pain syndrome: A case control study [abstract]. Arch Phys Med Rehabil, in press
3. Anderson J, Kaplan M: Brain injury obscured by chronic pain: A preliminary report. Arch Phys Med Rehabil 71:703–708, 1990
4. Andy OJ: Post-concussion syndrome: Brainstem seizures. A Case Report. Clin Electroencephalogr 20:24–34, 1989
5. Barth JT, Macciocchi SN, Ciordani B, et al: Neuropsychological sequelae of minor head injury. Neurosurgery 13:529–532, 1983
6. Binder LM: Malingering following minor head trauma. Clinical Neuropsychologist 4:25–36, 1990
7. Bonica JJ: The Management of Pain, ed 2, vol 1. Philadelphia, Lea & Febiger, 1990

8. Boquet J, Moore N, Boismare F, et al: Vertigo in post-concussional and migrainous patients: Implication of the autonomic nervous system. Agressologie 24:235–236, 1983
9. Braaf MM, Rosner S: Symptomatology and treatment of injured of the neck. NY State J Med 5:237–242, 1955
10. Brandt SA, Livingston A: Receptor changes in the spinal cord of sheep associated with exposure to chronic pain. Pain 42:323–329, 1990
11. Diamond S: Depression and headache. Headache 23:122–126, 1983
12. Dickmen S, McLean A, Temkin N: Neuropsychological and psychosocial consequences of minor head injury. J Neurol Neurosurg Psychiatry 49:1227–1232, 1986
13. Dickmen S, Reitan RM, Temkin NR: Neuropsychological recovery in head injury. Arch Neurol 40:333–338, 1983
14. Dubner R: Hyperalgesia and expanded receptive fields. Pain 48:3–4, 1992
15. Elkind AH: Headache and head trauma. Clinical Journal of Pain 5:77–87, 1989
16. Elkind AH: Headache and facial pain associated with head injury. Otolaryngol Clin North Am 22:1251–1271, 1989
17. Fedoroff JP, Starkstein SE, Forrester AW, et al: Depression in patients with acute traumatic brain injury. Am J Psychiatry 149:918–923, 1992
18. Fordyce WE, Roberts AH, Sternbach RA: The behavioral management of chronic pain: A Response to critics. Pain 22:113–125, 1985
19. Gibson SJ, Le Vasseur SA, Helme RD: Cerebral event–related responses induced by CO_2 laser stimulation in subjects suffering from cervico-brachial syndrome. Pain 47:173–182, 1991
20. Gronwall D, Wrightson P: Delayed recovery of intellectual function after minor head injury. Lancet 2:605–609, 1974
21. Gronwall D, Wrightson P: Cumulative effect of concussion. Lancet 2:995–997, 1975
22. Haas DC, Lourie H: Trauma-triggered migraine: An explanation for common neurological attacks after mild head injury. J Neurosurg 68:181–188, 1988
23. Hayes RL, Povlishock JT, Singha B: Pathophysiology of mild head injury. Physical Medicine & Rehabilitation: State of the Art Reviews 6:9–20, 1992
24. Hinoki M: Otoneurological observations on whiplash injuries to neck with special reference to the formation of equilibrial disorder. Clinical Surgery (Tokyo) 22:1683–1690, 1967
25. Hinoki M: Vertigo due to whiplash injury: A neurotological approach. Acta Otolaryngol Suppl (Stockh) 419:9–29, 1985
26. Horn LJ: Post-concussive headache. Physical Medicine & Rehabilitation: State of the Art Reviews 6:69–78, 1992
27. Jane JA, Steward O, Gennarelli T: Axonal degeneration induced by experimental non-invasive minor head injury. J Neurosurg 62:96–100, 1985
28. Jensen MP, Turner JA, Romano JM, et al: Coping with chronic pain: A critical review of the literature. Pain 47:249–283, 1991
29. Jensen OK, Nielson FF, Vosmar L: An open study comparing manual therapy with the use of cold packs in the treatment of post-traumatic headache. Cephalalgia 10:241–250, 1990
30. Kay T: Neuropsychological diagnosis: Disentangling the multiple determinants of functional disability after mild traumatic brain injury. Physical Medicine & Rehabilitation: State of the Art Reviews 6:109–127, 1992
31. Kelly R: The post traumatic syndrome: An Iatrogenic disease. Forensic Sci 6:17–24, 1975
32. Kewman DG, Vaishampayan N: Cognitive deficits in musculoskeletal pain patients. Arch Phys Med Rehabil 70:A-19, 1989
33. Kottke FJ, Lehmann JF: Krusen's Handbook of Physical Medicine and Rehabilitation, ed 4. Philadelphia, WB Saunders, 1990
34. Lehmann JF, Boswell S, Price R, et al: Quantitative evaluation of sway as an indicator of functional balance in post-traumatic brain injury. Arch Phys Med Rehabil 71:955–962, 1990
35. Leigh RJ, Zee DS: The Neurology of Eye Movements, ed 2. Philadelphia, FA Davis, 1991, p 111
36. Leininger B, Gramling S, Farrell A, et al: Neuropsychological deficits in symptomatic minor head injury patients after concussion and mild concussion. J Neurol Neurosurg Psychiatry 53:293–296, 1990

36a. Levin HS, Mattis S, Ruff RM, et al: Neurobehavioral outcome following minor head injury: A three-center study. J Neurosurg 66:234–243, 1987

37. McMordie WR: Twenty-year follow-up of the prevailing opinion on the post-traumatic or post-concussional syndrome. Clinical Neuropsychologist 2:198–212, 1988

38. MacNab I: Acceleration injuries of the cervical spine. J Bone Joint Surg [Am] 46:1797–1799, 1964

39. MacNab I: The "whiplash syndrome." Orthop Clin North Am 2:389–403, 1971

40. Mateer CA: Systems of care for post-concussive syndrome. Physical Medicine & Rehabilitation: State of the Art Reviews 6:143–160, 1992

41. Miller H: Accident neurosis. Br Med J 1:919, 1961

42. Miller L: Chronic pain complicating head injury recovery: Recommendations for clinicians. Cognitive Rehabilitation. (September/October):12–19, 1990

43. Oates J: Post-concussive balance dysfunction: A physical therapy approach. Physical Medicine & Rehabilitation: State of the Art Reviews 6:89–108, 1992

43a. Ommaya AK: The neck: Classification, physiology and clinical outcome of injuries to the neck in motor vehicle accidents. In Aldeman B, Chapon A (eds): Biomechanics of Impact Trauma. Amsterdam, Elsevier, 1984

44. Povlishock J, Becker D: Fate of reactive axonal swellings induced by head injury. Lab Invest 52:540–552, 1985

45. Povlishock J, Becker D, Cheng C, et al: Axonal change in minor head injury. J Neuropathol Exp Neurol 42:225–242, 1983

46. Reicke N: Der vertebrogene Schwindel: Aetiologie und Differntialdiagnose. Fortschr Med 96:1895–1902, 1978

47. Reik L: Cluster headache after head injury. Headache 27:509–510, 1987

48. Rimel R, Giordani B, Barth J, et al: Disability caused by minor head injury. Neurosurgery 9:221–228, 1981

49. Rutherford WH, Merrett JD, McDonald JR: Symptoms at one year following concussion from minor head injuries. Injury 10:225–230, 1979

50. Schoenen J, Bottin D, Hardy F, et al: Cephalic and extracephalic pressure pain thresholds in chronic tension-type headache. Pain 47:145–149, 1991

51. Sortland O, Tysvaie AT: Brain damage in former association football players. Neuroradiology 31:44–48, 1989

52. Travell JG, Simons DG: Myofascial Pain and Dysfunction: The Trigger Point Manual. Baltimore, Williams & Wilkins, 1983

53. Tysvaer AT, Storli OV, Bachen NI: Soccer injuries to the brain: A neurological and electroencephalographic study of former players. Acta Neurol Scand 80:151–158, 1989

54. Uomoto J, Esselman P: Traumatic brain injury and chronic pain: Differential types and rates by head injury severity. Arch Phys Med Rehabil in press

54a. Vernon H (ed): Upper Cervical Syndrome: Chiropractic Diagnosis and Treatment. Baltimore, Williams and Wilkins, 1988

54b. Whyte J, Rosenthal M: Rehabilitation of the patient with head injury. In Delisa JA (ed): Rehabilitation Medicine: Principles and Practice. Philadelphia, JB Lippincott, 1988

55. Wrightson P, Gronwall D: Time off work and symptoms after minor head injury. Injury 12:445–454, 1981

56. Yarnell PR, Rossie GV: Minor whiplash head injury with major debilitation. Brain Inj 2:255–258, 1988

57. Zasler N: Neuromedical diagnosis and management of post-concussive disorders. Physical Medicine & Rehabilitation: State of the Art Reviews 6:33–67, 1992

58. Zoltan B: Visual, visual-perceptual, and perceptual-motor deficits in brain-injured adults: Evaluation, treatment, and functional implications. Physical Medicine and Rehabilitation Clinics of North America 3:337–354, 1992

Address reprint requests to

Michael T. Andary, MD
Department of Physical Medicine and Rehabilitation
Michigan State University College of Osteopathic Medicine
B-401 West Fee Hall
East Lansing, MI 48824-1316

1047–9651/93 $0.00 + .20

THE MYTHOLOGY OF REFLEX SYMPATHETIC DYSTROPHY AND SYMPATHETICALLY MAINTAINED PAINS

José L. Ochoa, MD, PhD, DSc, and Renato J. Verdugo, MD

> Man will occasionally stumble over the truth, but most of the time
> he will pick himself up and continue on.
>
> WINSTON S. CHURCHILL

BACKGROUND

The term *reflex sympathetic dystrophy* (RSD) is commonly applied to the condition in patients who express chronic spontaneous pains associated with combinations of (1) various positive and negative sensory and motor phenomena (hypoesthesias, hyperalgesias, muscle weakness and spasms); (2) changes in color, temperature, or trophism of the symptomatic parts; and (3) subjective benefit from diagnostic or therapeutic sympathetic blocks, typically on a transient basis.

This diagnostic term is commonly thought to carry a number of connotations:

The physiology of the sympathetic system is deranged, as apparently documented by vasomotor changes.

The sympathetic system is a key determinant of the spontaneous pains and also of the accompanying positive or negative sensorimotor manifestations, the dystrophic changes, and, naturally, of the "autonomic" changes.

Sympathetic blocks would establish the diagnosis and, if performed repetitively, might eventually cure.

Sympathectomy usually cures the condition.

From Good Samaritan Hospital and Medical Center and Oregon Health Sciences
University, Portland, Oregon

PHYSICAL MEDICINE AND REHABILITATION CLINICS
OF NORTH AMERICA

151

The concept of RSD is also automatically associated with the history of pain science: the American Civil War and Weir Mitchell; René Leriche, World War I and sympathectomy; the Briton Peter W. Nathan and his brilliant sequence of ever-maturing concepts; and another Briton, Hannington-Kiff, and his regional intravenous sympathetic blocks. This association with history decorates the concept of RSD with solemn endorsements.

The ideas on RSD became cleverly updated when basic scientists working on animal experimental aspects of human painful syndromes took an interest not only in physiologic and pathologic relationships between the sympathetic and the afferent systems but also in matters of clinical expertise. For example, W.J. Roberts emphasized that sympathetic discharge may activate low-threshold tactile sensory units in limbs of animals. Roberts reasoned that sympathetic outflow might trigger tactile sensory input in humans. If central neurons capable of evoking pain were to become abnormally sensitized in patients, primary sensory information from tactile afferent units would evoke pain. Such pain would occur in response to normally innocuous tactile stimulation (hyperalgesia, allodynia) or would be determined by tonic or phasic sympathetic efferent discharge, giving rise to an apparently spontaneous sympathetically maintained pain.[41] *Sympathetically maintained pain* (SMP) was defined by Roberts as "characterized by: a) a history of physical trauma on the painful area; b) the presence of a continuous burning pain together with mechanical hyperalgesia/allodynia (painful sensation to touch); and c) relief from the pain during sympathetic block." *Sympathetically independent pain* is the term used by others to define the pain of patients who do not respond to blocks.[12, 50]

Jänig, a distinguished scientist from Kiel and an authority on physiology of the sympathetic system, has launched emphatic attempts at understanding the interface between normal and abnormal physiology of the sympathetic system and the clinical condition RSD.[17] Other renowned scientists from the National Institutes of Health in Bethesda, Maryland, have generated a powerful animal model of painful nerve injury that has yielded important data on basic mechanisms, the assessment of which requires invasive approaches inapplicable to the human patient.[3] The realization that these nerve-injured animals display pain behavior, hyperalgesias, vasomotor phenomena, and even dystrophic changes in the symptomatic limbs renders them at first sight as irresistible animal models of RSD. For some researchers, these animals serve as appropriate models of SMP, too, because their painful behavior would be abolished by suppressing sympathetic outflow to the affected limb.[19, 48] For other researchers, they would not quite amount to models of SMP.[14]

DIAGNOSTIC TERMS: RSD AND RELATED CONDITIONS

The official definition of RSD by the International Association for the Study of Pain (IASP)[16] can be abbreviated as follows:

Continuous pain in a portion of an extremity after trauma which may include fracture but *does not involve a major nerve*, associated with *sympathetic hyperactivity* . . . The pain is described as burning, continuous, exacerbated by movement, cutaneous stimulation, or stress. [The onset is] usually weeks after injury. Associated symptoms [include the presence of] initial vaso-dilatation with increasing temperature, hyperhidrosis and oedema. Hyperhidrosis and reduced sympathetic activity may also occur. Atrophy of skin appendages, cool, red, and clammy skin are variably present. Disuse atrophy of deep structures may progress to Sudeck's atrophy of bone. Aggravated by use of the body part, and relieved by immobilization . . . Later vasospastic symptoms become prominent with persistent coldness of the affected extremity, pallor and cyanosis, atrophy of the skin and nails, loss of hair, atrophy of soft tissues and stiffness of joints. Without therapy these symptoms may persist. It is not necessary for one patient to exhibit all symptoms together. An additional limb or limbs may be affected as well.

The "signs" are described by the IASP as "variable. . . . There may be florid signs of sympathetic hyperactivity." As "laboratory findings . . . in advanced cases, roentgenogram may show atrophy of bone." The "usual course" is characterized as follows: "persists indefinitely if untreated, with a small incidence of spontaneous remission. *Relief: Sympathetic block and physical therapy; sympathectomy if long-term results are not achieved with repeated blocks;* may respond in early phases to high doses of corticosteroids, e.g., prednisone 50 mg daily."

It is appropriate to wonder why this definition of RSD is so readily associated with Weir Mitchell. That distinguished author coined the term *causalgia* (burning pain) to describe the painful syndrome his soldiers expressed after nerve injury. Mitchell certainly did not use the term RSD as a diagnostic category for his patients, and although today he would have been an outcast by failing to diagnose RSD in those patients, as explained later, Mitchell did not neglect consideration of the sympathetic system in his hypothesis about pathophysiologic mechanisms in causalgia. In fact, pioneer authors who published ideas and observations on painful syndromes that fit today's criteria for RSD uniformly talked about causalgia. The term RSD only pervaded the literature in the 1950s to define a clinical condition that is retrospectively inseparable from classic causalgia. In facing this taxonomic issue, the IASP arbitrated that although in causalgia there is clear nerve injury, in RSD there is none, but the symptoms are grossly the same.

The IASP[16] defines causalgia in these terms: "Burning pain, allodynia, and hyperpathia, usually in the hand or foot, *after partial injury of a nerve or one of its major branches . . .* Onset usually immediately after partial nerve injury or, may be delayed for months. "Causalgia" of the radial nerve is very rare. The nerves most commonly involved are the median, the sciatic and tibial, and ulnar. Spontaneous pain. Pain described as constant, burning; exacerbated by light touch, stress, temperature change, movement of the involved limb, visual and auditory stimuli, e.g., a sudden sound or bright light, emotional disturbance." The "associated symptoms" descibed are "atrophy of skin appendages, secondary atrophic changes in bones, joints and muscles; cool, reddish, clammy skin with excessive sweating; sensory and motor loss in structures innervated by the damaged portion of nerve." The "laboratory findings" mentioned by the IASP include "galvanic skin responses and plethysmography reveal[ing] *signs of sympathetic nervous system hyperactivity.* Roentgenogram may show atrophy of bone. . . . If untreated, the majority of patients will have symptoms which persist indefinitely; spontaneous remission occurs. Relief: In early stages of "Causalgia" (first few months) sympathetic blockade plus vigorous physical therapy usually provides transient relief; *repeated blocks usually lead to long-term relief. When a series of sympathetic blocks does not provide long-term relief, sympathectomy is indicated.* Long-term persistence of symptoms reduces the likelihood of successful therapy."

Ambiguities surrounding the concepts of RSD and causalgia, now obvious to the reader, have also become obvious to a group of scientists and clinicians who recently authored a compromise definition[18]: "RSD is a descriptive term meaning a *complex disorder or a group of disorders* that may develop *as a consequence of trauma* affecting the limbs, *with or without an obvious nerve lesion. . . .* It consists of *pain and related sensory abnormalities, abnormal blood flow* and sweating, *abnormalities in the motor system* and changes in structure of both superficial and deep tissues. . . . It is agreed that the name reflex sympathetic dystrophy is used in a descriptive sense and *does not imply specific underlying mechanisms."*

This Consensus Statement by Jänig et al in 1991 becomes overly conservative to the point that neither an underlying mechanism nor a specific therapy is put forth. This point of view is commendable in its rigor but has the semantic drawback that, in its diffuseness, it spares few neurologic conditions associated with pain. This definition of RSD nearly equals "painful symptoms following a health problem." Thus, the reader no longer asks what is RSD but wonders what is not RSD. A logistic danger is that, despite bland unspecificity, this Consensus Definition,[18] which defuses RSD, keeps the word sympathetic in it. Under the protection of this definition, now there need be no constraint in targeting "therapy" against the sympathetic for any assortment of pains associated with combinations of motor, sensory, or neurovascular symptoms. Moreover, physicians crusading against RSD are now given a colossal work overload.[38]

It thus becomes imperative to emphasize that RSD is a diagnosis. RSD is not a *disease,* because there is no particular cause for it. Moreover, it is not a *syndrome,* because there is no single pathophysiologic mechanism behind it. RSD is a *symptom complex* underlain by any of several possible pathophysiologic mechanisms, in turn caused by any of many possible factors. From a broad personal experience, the symptom complex of RSD may be expressed in connection with any of multiple documented syndromes: sensitized primary nociceptors; bona fide injury to peripheral nervous system at roots, plexus, or peripheral nerves; spinal cord lesions; injuries to the encephalon; hysteria and related psychiatric disorders; Munchausen's syndrome; malingering; or combinations thereof.

CRITIQUE

Historical Aspects

The historical trajectory of concepts pertaining to the role of the sympathetic system in chronic pain has been deformed by recitation of citations.[38] It is shocking to realize that Mitchell rejected the idea that causalgia, an all-embracing term in his time, was related to the sympathetic system. For Mitchell,[31] "nerves are usually divided into those known as cerebro-spinal and those belonging to the great sympathetic system. The former chiefly concern at present, since, indeed, the later are rarely injured, and since their disease have only of late begun to claim attention."

In turn, Leriche's[23] Corporal G., who had a severe neurovascular lesion at left retroclavicular level, did not have RSD by current IASP criteria: what Leriche severed for therapy was the perivascular sympathetic innervation of his patient's humeral artery, and what he apparently improved were probably ischemic ulcers, not neuropathic pain.[38] Thoughtful Dr. W. K. Livingston [28] had more solid arguments than Mitchell in concluding that ". . . one might start by abandoning, for the time being, the assumption that the activities of the sympathetic nerves represent the essential factor in either the cause or the cure of the causalgic syndrome." It is disconcerting to the reader that, today, Dr. J. Hannington-Kiff, the author who introduced guanethidine regional sympathetic blocks for RSD, believes that it is not through abolition of sympathetic function that sympathetic blocks transiently relieve the condition.[15, 35]

Vasomotor Phenomena

Vasomotor dysfunction is unquestionably the mechanism behind the changes in color and temperature observed in symptomatic RSD skin. This finding may certainly be of sympathetic origin; however, the vasomotor deviations, particularly in the direction of hyperthermia, may be strictly unrelated to function or dysfunction of the sympathetic system and instead due to nociceptor-mediated antidromic vasodilatation determined by neurosecretion of vasoactive substances.[25, 32] When legitimately autonomic in origin, vasomotor changes might simply be a natural reflex response to anomalous sensory input rather than an abnormal state of the sympathetic system[2, 33] or may be generated in the brain through biofeedback mechanism. Signs of "exaggerated sympathetic activity" might even be a consequence of sympathetic denervation supersensitivity, as reported before[26, 33] and as recently postulated by Drummond et al,[10] who have found diminished concentration of noradrenaline and its metabolite 3,4-dihydroxyphenylethyleneglycol in extremities with RSD. To the embarrassment of medical practice, some of these patients are equivocally condemned to sympathectomy. Whatever the mechanism behind the vasomotor changes, engagement of the sympathetic system in the generation of vasomotor changes in symptomatic limbs in RSD does not mean that the sympathetic is necessarily involved in the generation of pain.[33–36, 38]

Dystrophy

Regressive dystrophic changes in causalgia-RSD-SMP may sometimes occur when the symptomatic limb harbors a genuine neurologic injury.[5, 43] Dystrophy may even develop after sympathectomy. Disuse may, by itself, cause profound changes in muscle and skin, particularly at dependent body parts. Although bony changes are nonspecific,[49] they have been assumed to be characteristic of RSD.[20] The ligature sign, featuring a sharp boundary of distal edema in a limb and proposed by Schwartzman[45] as a pathognomonic sign of RSD, is intriguing. A case of Munchausen's syndrome understandably had edema, and even "classic bone scan findings" of RSD, after self-inflicted ligature.[42] It must be stressed that only a minority of patients with RSD display dystrophic changes in the absence of nerve injury. We have come across several remarkable examples of patients with mysterious RSD and marked swelling, pigmentation, or infection of the symptomatic limb. In them, we have characteristically found evidence of absence of pertinent organic neurologic dysfunction, explicit evidence that the motor and sensory deficits are psychogenic in origin, and separate evidence of crippling psychiatric pathology.

Dystonia

We have yet to come across a patient with RSD and dystonia, or muscle spasms, who is eventually proven to have a satisfactory organic basis for the painful syndrome and sensorimotor phenomena. Basal ganglia experts continue to puzzle about this enigma.[22, 29, 46]

Sympathectomy

Outcome studies on the effect of sympathectomy on these chronic painful syndromes are not available. The concept of cure of RSD by sympathectomy is fantastic. Sadly, basic scientists have taken the clinician's word for granted and have engaged in a "reciprocation of fantasy" cycle with clinicians on the role of the sympathetic system in chronic pains in patients.[35] Not only was Leriche often not quite dealing with RSD patients but he openly questioned the role of ablation of the sympathetic chain in the treatment of causalgia:

> Quite a considerable number of surgeons, especially in the United States, reject periarterial sympathectomy altogether on theoretical grounds. They continue to shut their eyes to the very numerous positive achievements to the credit of this operation, and they do far too many useless ganglionectomies. And at the present time, with an experience of more than 1,200 sympathetic operations, I am of opinion that, in the case of causalgia, it is proper to begin always with a periarterial operation, carried out at an appropriate level. If it should fail, there will still be time to consider whether one should attack the ganglionic chain. But I have the impression that, in the cases of which I am speaking, when there is neither vascular lesion nor lesion of a nerve trunk, if the periarterial operation has been a failure, it is not at all likely that an operation on the ganglia will achieve any greater success.[24]

> For Leriche,[23] "le traitement de ces algies vaso-motrices consiste peut-être à modifier l'innervation sympathique pervertie en agissant sur les plexus nerveux péri-artériels que l'on suppose intéressés. Pour cela, il faut exciser la gaine celluleuse péri-artérielle sur une certaine étendue (8 à 10 cm.) [the treatment of these vasomotor pains perhaps consists of modifying the altered sympathetic innervation by operating on the periarterial nerve plexus that are believed involved. For this, it is necessary to cut off the periarterial cellulous sheath to a certain length (8 to 10 cm)—editor's translation]."

We were taught a sobering lesson by the last patient we condemned to sympathectomy, a young man who had a full-blown syndrome of RSD-SMP after physical trauma. There were clear-cut abnormalities in the thermal emission profile of the symptomatic limb, detected by thermography. The patient expressed mechanical and thermal hyperalgesia, measured quantitatively by algometry and the Marstock thermotest method. He responded encouragingly to sympathetic blocks, on a transient basis, and underwent upper thoracic sympathectomy performed by a skilled neurosurgeon. He was cured for 2 months. Then, the syndrome reappeared, the same as before sympathectomy. Sympathectomy had been physiologically effective, as documented by postoperative sympathetic function parameters. The anesthesiologist was then asked to attempt a paravertebral block. After local anesthetic block, pain and hyperalgesia disappeared totally for a whole week. When the patient requested another block, we administered an injection of saline near the surgical scar, and the painful syndrome was again cured for a whole week. He called again, and the placebo injection was repeated on another two occasions, with the same rewarding outcome.

Sympathetic Blocks

RSD is not cured by sympathetic blocks. This opinion is shared by a patient who had more than 60 sympathetic blocks and three sympathectomies to different limbs.[35] Another patient, an unfortunate professional musician from New York who has had more than 100 blocks for RSD of the left arm, also witnesses this kind of failure. Amputation is now being considered to relieve her pain.

Somehow, we have succumbed to the belief that sympathetic blocks might cure. Our profession will forever remain embarrassed about the naiveté of adjudicating diagnostic and pathophysiologic meaning to the patient's subjective response during the ritualistic medical intervention constituting a "diagnostic" sympathetic block. Should the patient volunteer subjective improvement, the doctor will issue a confident diagnosis, assume specific pathophysiology, and condemn the patient to perpetual blocks and eventual sympathectomy. These initiatives are characteristically doomed to failure. Remorse for our simple-mindedness about such diagnostic criterion is compounded by stupefied aware-ness that world-reputed series of diagnostic sympathetic blocks, from several countries, have been placebo uncontrolled.[34, 35] When placebo control is imple-mented, it is found that the active drug really works no better than placebo.[13, 52]

The misleading repercussions on medical practice of universal nonchalance with non–placebo-controlled sympathetic blocks are multiplied by virtue of the fact that patients expressing chronic painful syndromes classifiable as RSD have an inordinately high incidence of placebo response (Verdugo and Ochoa, sub-mitted for publication, 1992).[51] It cannot be seen lightheartedly that the 10% incidence of assessed placebo responders within the RSD population reported by Raja et al[40] is less than one third the rate of placebo responders (36%) in the general population[11] and is about one sixth the rate found in a much larger population of chronic "neuropathic" pain patients.[51] These low percentages question stringency of the placebo control paradigm.[34, 35, 38]

Phentolamine Blocks and SMP

The idea that phentolamine blocks diagnose SMP involves circular argu-ment: Roberts[41] defines SMP as "pain relieved during sympathetic block," and Raja et al[40] state that sympathetic block with phentolamine is "a diagnostic test for sympathetically maintained pain."

It has been remarked that "sympathetically maintained pain appears to be a condition wherein pain is related to activation of peripheral α-adrenergic recep-tors."[40] A phentolamine test was used by Olsson et al[39] in 79 girls and 6 boys with reflex sympathetic dystrophy, and Arnér[1] recently published results on 48 adults and 56 children; however, Olsson et al[39] did not perform placebo control, and Arnér controlled for placebo in only an unspecified percentage of his adult patients. In turn, "one or more boluses of 3–5 ml. normal saline were adminis-tered through the peripheral IV line as a placebo" by Raja et al.[40]

The quality of the pharmacologic species administered in sympathetic blocks is of little relevance in terms of pain response. This by itself questions the nature of the response to sympathetic blocks. Indeed, Hannington-Kiff[15, 35] now claims that injection of morphine into sympathetic ganglia relieves pain better than sympathetic blocks, even though morphine does not block sympathetic function. For Glynn, this effect is just the specific analgesic action of slowly released morphine. Glynn also finds that inert placebo substances may be as successful as guanethidine or even phentolamine.[35, 38]

The Clonidine Patch Test

"The concept that spontaneous pain (directly) and hyperalgesia (indirectly) in 'RSD-SMP' are mediated by anomalous insertion of alpha adrenergic recep-tors in primary nociceptors, has been apparently boosted by the observation that application of a Clonidine patch to 'SMP' skin relieved pain evoked by me-chanical and cold stimuli hyperalgesia in one patient with a sciatic nerve in-jury diagnosed as having 'SMP', based on lumbar sympathetic blockade." Since this statement by Ochoa and Verdugo about the communication by Davis et al[8, 38] the observation has been extended by Davis and colleagues[9] to new patients.

However, Glynn and Jones[13] tested oral clonidine, as well as local Bier block, using clonidine in 22 patients. They concluded that "clonidine appears to have provided effective sympathetic blockade as measured by the diminished vaso-constrictor ice response, but without better analgesia when compared to placebo injection," raising "some questions in explanation of the peripheral mechanisms of RSD."

It would seem advisable to revise the evidence on the clonidine patch test before becoming carried away by its apparent pathophysiologic appeal.

PLACEBO EFFECTS

The few studies that have included rigorous placebo control for diagnostic blocks have reached the conclusion that sympathetic blockade is not convincingly better than placebo in producing analgesia. This score is even more categoric because it must be corrected for the phenomenon of *active* placebo effect exerted by active agents, which leads to overestimation of specific drug effect.

Important nuances of placebo response and its control and assessment are exemplified in the case of a patient who was rigorously studied, initially by Dr. James Campbell's group in Maryland, then by our team in Portland, and then again in Maryland. The two groups reached diametrically opposed conclusions, although they were mutually aware of each other's views. For Campbell et al,[4] this unfortunate patient has SMP due to pathologic activation of peripheral α-adrenergic receptors and is not a placebo responder. For the Maryland group, the patient carries an organic neurologic disorder that antedated multiple failed oral surgical and neurosurgical procedures, inclusive of a nerve graft that con-fused the clinical picture.[4] For the Portland group, the patient suffers from a primary psychological disorder associated with somatization, as lucidly de-scribed in modern terms by Lipowski.[27] In Portland, her response to phentol-amine block was obviously placebo effect.[52]

Placebo effect is certainly underestimated.[7] Can it be overestimated? If so, nonplacebo responders with potential SMP should be relieved by sympathetic blocks. We have never seen this as a legitimate result in a population of close to 60 nonresponders tested with phentolamine (Verdugo et al, submitted for pub-lication, 1992).[52]

MASTER OPINIONS ON RSD

How often is a disappointed practitioner frank enough to publish his subsequent disenchantment? Perhaps editorial waiting lists are too long for disconcerting disclaimers. Surely there is room for a *Journal of Fatuous Findings,* a *Revue de Neurologie Manqué.* Such periodicals would be a worthy vehicle for those would-be Marco Polos of neurology who imagine they have stumbled upon some novel syndrome or a physical sign fit to be mentioned in the same breath as the Babinski phenomenon. These preliminary and cynical reflections encourage one to ventilate a long-projected idea of expressing certain doubts about the status of a number of neurological fancies which smack more romance than reason.[6]

One frank practitioner forwarded the following personal communication:

Geoff Schott and I have belatedly come to the conclusion that no results which are not controlled by saline injection should be accepted for publication. We have seen this as-tounding phenomenon—a patient who will not allow you to touch his limb and lo and behold! you can do what you like with it after intravenous saline. Research should be on how to learn what people do to achieve a placebo effect. Some people can do it easily, others not. I once wrote a letter (with Prof. Watson of Barts) to the *Lancet* saying that the placebo effect was the pharmacologist's enemy but the doctor's friend. Unfortunately medical students are taught by pharmacologists. *Presumably our two discoveries:* a) Pain is removed even if it arises above the cuff, by guanethidine injected below the cuff, and b) pain arising in the CNS as thalamic syndrome is also sometimes relieved by guanethidine, *are placebo effects.* (Nathan PW: personal communication, June 15, 1991.)

ANIMAL MODELS

The scientific rationale underlying the concepts of RSD and SMP is questionable. There are excellent animal models of nerve or root injury causing equivalents of causalgia.[3, 19, 44, 47]; however, there is weak evidence that they may provide legitimate models of human RSD or SMP. Chronic pain after nerve injury in humans is relatively rare.[34] Thus, the multiple primary peripheral and secondary central nervous system abnormalities consistently demonstrated after experimental nerve injury in animals must include epiphenomena probably inadequate to explain the inconsistent and multifaceted human pain syndromes. The specific pathology and pathophysiology underlying animal nerve injury models are unlikely to represent the universal pathology and pathophysiology of human RSD. In other words, to the extent they involve nerve injury, animal models of "Reflex Sympathetic Dystrophy and related syndromes"[17] are excellent models of just that—nerve injury—and, when leading to pain, are surrogate models of causalgia. These logical animal preparations are poor and misleading models for the concrete entity SMP and for the magical entity RSD. The human model of human painful nerve injury, the human model of SMP, and the human model of RSD, when professionally evaluated without bias or mystification, are the best models of all. Provisos such as "animal behavior which might be indicative of . . ."[17] just do not apply to human models. That is why Jänig's edict[17] "what should be done #3: Components . . . of the RSD syndrome should be tested in animal model experimentation in vivo and in vitro . . ." is a flaw of experimental design.

There are no authentic animal models for RSD. Given the all-embracing consensus definition of RSD by Jänig et al,[18] it would be surprising if a unitary pathophysiologic animal model could be found for that diffuse complex that represents multiple possible pathophysiologies. Moreover, to the extent that psychological mechanisms are so intrinsic to some of the human conditions, it is hard to conceive of an appropriate animal model for them.

WHAT NEUROLOGISTS FIND RSD PATIENTS TO HAVE

Patients expressing chronic painful states classifiable under the symptom complex RSD are usually managed with bypassing of neurologic evaluation.[37]

These patients break down into multiple disparate pathophysiologic categories when tested rigorously for clinical, neurophysiologic, pharmacologic, and psychophysical parameters. The major subgroups are

   Primary organic disease of the nervous system that explains the whole syndrome
   Hysteria, conversion, and somatization that explains the whole syndrome—this diagnosis is usually missed before neurologic and psychiatric evaluation

Mixed cases, which prove most challenging from the diagnostic point of view.

Disappointingly, a sizable school of psychiatrists tends to conclude compulsively that, in a patient with RSD and psychiatric dysfunction, the former has caused the latter. Fortunately, among academic psychiatrists the issue still remains controversial.[30, 53] In practice, at the stage of *diagnosis*, these specialists are reserved a passive role because, although their expertise can rule in psychological dysfunction, it does not rule out possibly coexistent organic dysfunction sufficient to legitimately cause a chronic painful syndrome. In addition, these specialists are not equipped to pinpoint psychogenicity as the basis of apparently authentic positive and negative motor and sensory neuromuscular symptoms due in reality to somatization. This can be explicitly documented by informed neurologists.[34, 35]

Ultimately, psychiatrists and psychologists have a key role in *management* of many of these patients. Although many patients resist the idea, we have seen astonishing cures of chronic RSD patients who had no evidence of organic neurologic disease (other than iatrogenic autonomic failure) cured by expert psychiatric management (by Stinnett in Philadelphia and Rosenbaum in Portland).

We have studied several hundred patients rigorously through multidisciplinary approaches, including some invasive methods often used in animal experimentation. The majority of patients with RSD in the civilian population either have no organic cause for their apparently neurologic syndrome or have a nerve injury that has been complicated by psychogenic overlay.

A DANGEROUS DIAGNOSIS

RSD is not a *disease* nor a *syndrome* but is just a *symptom complex* that carries the illusion of a defined pathophysiology. The illusion in turn triggers programmed diagnostic testing and programmed treatment. The diagnostic test is an embarrassing misunderstanding. Treatment through sympathectomy fails. RSD is a dangerous diagnosis, because patients may be hurt by omission of a true pathophysiologic diagnosis for their symptom complex, and by commission through unnecessary, expensive, and often mutilating therapies. This dangerous diagnosis has been made even more dangerous, as mentioned earlier, by introduction of an all-embracing definition that unfortunately retains the word *sympathetic*. Now, any well-intended practitioner can believe himself or herself entitled to issue this mythical diagnosis and to condemn patients to its consequences.[38]

Keeping in mind that some of the concepts that we have expressed here are probably correct, it becomes an obligation for the scientist and the clinician to consider these ideas during fair self-assessment of theoretic rationales and management rituals on RSD. This will be most difficult for minorities with vested clinical or research interests in perpetuating the concept that the sympathetic system is, in one way or another, instrumental in determining a chronic neurologic syndrome in patients who, bluntly speaking, are assessed through double medical-scientific standards. The time for a paradigm shift, á la Kuhn,[21] is ripe for the myth of RSD.

References

1. Arnér S: Intravenous phentolamine test: Diagnostic and prognostic use in reflex sympathetic dystrophy. Pain 46:17–22, 1991

2. Bennett GJ, Ochoa JL: Thermographic observations on rats with experimental neuropathic pain. Pain 45:61–67, 1991
3. Bennett GJ, Xie Y-K: A peripheral mononeuropathy in rat that produces disorders of pain sensation like those seen in man. Pain 33:87–107, 1988
4. Campbell JN, Raja SN, Meyer RA: How should sympathetically maintained pain be diagnosed? A case study. In Besson JM, Guilbaud G (eds): Lesions of Primary Afferent Fibers as a Tool for the Study of Clinical Pain. Amsterdam, Elsevier, 1991, pp 45–51
5. Cline MA, Ochoa J, Torebjörk HE: Chronic hyperalgesia and skin warming caused by sensitized C nociceptors. Brain 112:621–647, Figure 1, 1989
6. Critchley M: Mythical maladies of the nervous system. In The Citadel of the Senses and Other Essays. New York, Raven Press, 1986, p 85
7. Davis JM: Don't let placebos fool you. Postgrad Med 88:21–24, 1990
8. Davis KD, Campbell JN, Raja SN, et al: Topical application of an α_2-adrenergic agonist relieves hyperalgesia in sympathetically maintained pain. Pain Suppl S:S421, 1990
9. Davis KD, Treede RD, Raja SN, et al: Topical application of clonidine relieves hyperalgesia in patients with sympathetically maintained pain. Pain 47:309–317, 1991
10. Drummond PD, Finch PM, Smythe GA: Reflex sympathetic dystrophy: The significance of differing plasma catecholamine concentrations in affected and unaffected limbs. Brain 114:2025–2036, 1991
11. Evans FJ: The placebo response in pain reduction. Adv Neurol 4:289–296, 1974
12. Frost SA, Raja SN, Campbell JN, et al: Does hyperalgesia to cooling stimuli characterize patients with sympathetically maintained pain (reflex sympathetic dystrophy)? In Dubner R, Gebhart GF, Bond MR (eds): Proceedings of the Vth World Congress on Pain, Pain Research and Clinical Management. Amsterdam, Elsevier, 1988, pp 151–156
13. Glynn C, Jones P: An investigation of the role of clonidine in the treatment of reflex sympathetic dystrophy. In Stanton-Hicks M, Jänig W, Boas R (eds): Reflex Sympathetic Dystrophy. Boston, Kluwer, 1989, pp 187–196
14. Guilbaud G: Some electrophysiological and pharmacological aspects of primary and secondary distant hyperalgesia in mononeuropathic rats. In New Trends in Referred Pain and Hyperalgesia. University "G. D'Annunzio" International Congress. Chieti, Italy, 1992, p 31
15. Hannington-Kiff JG: Does failed natural opioid modulation in regional sympathetic ganglia cause reflex sympathetic dystrophy? Lancet 338:1125–1127, 1991
16. International Association for the Study of Pain: Classification of chronic pain: Descriptions of chronic pain syndromes and definitions of pain terms: Prepared by the Subcommittee on Taxonomy. Pain Suppl 3, 1986
17. Jänig W: Experimental approach to reflex sympathetic dystrophy and related syndromes. Pain 46:241–245, 1991
18. Jänig W, Blumberg H, Boas RA, et al: The reflex sympathetic dystrophy syndrome: Consensus statement and general recommendations for diagnosis and clinical research. In Bond MR, Charlton JE, Woolf CJ (eds): Proceedings of the VIth World Congress on Pain. Amsterdam, Elsevier, 1991, pp 373–376
19. Kim SH, Chung JM: Sympathectomy alleviates mechanical allodynia in an experimental animal model for neuropathy in the rat. Neurosci Lett 134:131–134, 1991
20. Kozin F, Genant HK, Bekerman C, et al: The reflex sympathetic dystrophy syndrome. II. Roentgenographic and scintigraphic evidence of bilaterality and of periarticular accentuation. Am J Med 60:332–338, 1976
21. Kuhn TS: The Structure of Scientific Revolutions, ed 2 enlarged. Chicago, University of Chicago Press, 1970
22. Lang A, Fahn S: Movement disorder of RSD. Neurology 40:1476–1477, 1990
23. Leriche R: De la Causalgie, envisagée comme une névrite du sympathique et de son traitement par la dénudation et l'excision des plexus nerveux péri-arteriels. Presse Med 24:178–180, 1916
24. Leriche R: The Surgery of Pain. Baltimore, Williams & Wilkins, 1939, pp 48–52
25. Lewis T: Vascular Disorders of the Limbs, Described for Practitioners and Students. London, Macmillan, 1936, p 93
26. Lindblom U, Ochoa JL: Somatosensory function and dysfunction. In Asbury AK,

McKhann GM, McDonald WI (eds): Disease of the Nervous System, vol II, ed 2. Philadelphia, WB Saunders, 1992, pp 213–228

27. Lipowski ZJ: Chronic idiopathic painful syndrome. Ann Med 22:213–217, 1990
28. Livingston WK: Pain Mechanisms. New York, Macmillan, 1947, p 215
29. Marsden CD, Obeso JA, Traub MM, et al: Muscle spasms associated with Sudeck's atrophy after injury. Br Med J 288:173–176, 1984
30. Merskey H: Regional pain is rarely hysterical. Arch Neurol 45:915–918, 1988
31. Mitchell SW: Injuries of Nerves and Their Consequences (1872). American Academy of Neurology Reprint Series. New York, Dover Publications, 1965
32. Ochoa JL: The newly recognized painful ABC syndrome: Thermographic aspects. Thermology 2:65–107, 1986
33. Ochoa JL: Neuropathic pains from within: Personal experiences, experiments and reflections on mythology. In Dimitrijevic R (ed): Altered Sensation and Pain. (Recent Achievements in Restorative Neurology, vol 3). Basel, S. Karger, 1989, pp 26–34
34. Ochoa JL: Afferent and sympathetic roles in chronic "neuropathic" pains: Confessions on misconceptions. In Besson JM, Guilbaud, G (eds): Lesions of Primary Afferent Fibers as a Tool for the Study of Clinical Pain. Amsterdam, Elsevier, 1991, pp 25–44
35. Ochoa JL: Controversies on chronic somatic pain and the sympathetic system: A five year chronicle. In Hamann W, Wedley JR (eds): Physiological Mechanisms of Pain and Pharmocology of Analgesia, April 1991. Guy's Hospital London, in press
36. Ochoa JL: A dangerous diagnosis to be given [editorial]. European Journal of Pain 12:63–64, 1991
37. Ochoa JL: Scientific clinical evaluation of chronic neuropathic painful syndromes. Presented at the American Academy of Neurology, Pain Annual Meeting Course 241. Payne R, Director, 1991, pp 15–31
38. Ochoa JL, Verdugo R: Reflex sympathetic dystrophy: Definitions and history of the ideas: A critical review of human studies. In Low PA (ed): The Evaluation and Management of Clinical Autonomic Disorders. Boston, Little, Brown, 1992
39. Olsson G, Arnér S, Hirsch G: Reflex sympathetic dystrophy in children. In Tyler DC, Krane EJ (eds): Pediatric Pain (Advances in Pain Research and Therapy, vol 15.) New York, Raven Press, 1990, pp 323–331
40. Raja SN, Treede R-D, Davis K, et al: Systemic alpha-adrenergic blockade with phentolamine: A diagnostic test for sympathetically maintained pain. Anesthesiology 74:691–698, 1991
41. Roberts WJ: A hypothesis on the physiological basis for causalgia and related pains. Pain 24:297–311, 1986
42. Rodríguez-Moreno J, Ruiz-Martin JM, Mateo-Soria L, et al: Munchausen's syndrome simulating reflex sympathetic dystrophy. Ann Rheum Dis 49:1010–1012, 1990
43. Rosenbaum RB, Ochoa JL: Carpal Tunnel Syndrome and Other Disorders of the Median Nerve. London, Butterworths, 1992, Figure 16–2
44. Sato J, Perl ER: Adrenergic excitation of cutaneous pain receptors induced by peripheral nerve injury. Science 251:1608–1610, 1991
45. Schwartzman RJ: Reflex sympathetic dystrophy: Concepts and controversies. Presented at the Tenth Annual Scientific Meeting, American Pain Society. New Orleans, November 7–10, 1991. Recorded by Sound Images, Inc., Aurora, CO (303–693-5511)
46. Schwartzman RJ, Kerrigan J: The movement disorder of reflex sympathetic dystrophy. Neurology 40:57–61, 1990
47. Seltzer Z, Dubner R, Shir Y: A novel behavioral model of neuropathic pain disorders produced by partial sciatic nerve injury in rats. Pain 43:205–218, 1990
48. Shir Y, Seltzer Z: Effects of sympathectomy in a model of causalgiform pain produced by partial sciatic nerve injury in rats. Pain 45:309–320, 1991
49. Steinert H, Nickel O, Hahn K: Three-phase bone scanning in reflex sympathetic dystrophy. In Stanton-Hicks M, Jänig W, Boas R (eds): Reflex Sympathetic Dystrophy. Boston, Kluwer, 1990
50. Treede R-D, Raja SN, Davis KD, et al: Evidence that peripheral alpha-adrenergic receptors mediate sympathetically maintained pain. In Bond MR, Charlton JE, Woolf CJ (eds): Proceedings of the VIth World Congress on Pain. Amsterdam, Elsevier, 1991, pp 377–382

51. Verdugo R, Ochoa JL: High incidence of placebo responders among chronic neuro-
    pathic pain patients. Ann Neurol 30:229, 1991
52. Verdugo R, Rosenblum S, Ochoa J: Phentolamine sympathetic blocks mislead diagno-
    sis. Soc Neurosci Abstr 17:107, 1991
53. Weintraub MI: Regional pain is usually hysterical. Arch Neurol 45:914–915, 1988

Address reprint requests to

José L. Ochoa, MD, PhD, DSc
Good Samaritan Hospital and Medical Center
1040 N.W. 22nd Avenue, Suite N460
Portland, OR 97210

TREATMENT APPROACHES TO REFLEX SYMPATHETIC DYSTROPHY

Michael C. Brody, MD, and Michael T. Andary, MD

Reflex sympathetic dystrophy (RSD) is a syndrome characterized by symptoms of sympathetic hyperactivity with relief of these clinical symptoms by interruption of the sympathetic innervation to the affected area. Because of the ambiguity of criteria used for the assessment of RSD and the lack of understanding of its pathophysiologic mechanisms, research attempting to define a rational approach of therapy is similarly enigmatic. Peer-reviewed articles describing approaches in the treatment of RSD are typically anecdotal and biased, consisting of case reports, retrospective reviews, or uncontrolled design. Given the limitations of available literature, we attempt herein to provide an overview of strategies that have been described to relieve the symptoms and minimize the progressive disability associated with RSD.

Unfortunately, the pain caused by RSD is only one of the problems faced by the patient and clinician. Other problems include vocational impairments, disability, psychological problems, and deconditioning complications. Treatment programs for patients with RSD should consider the following factors:

treatment or amelioration of the underlying precipitating cause of RSD (e.g., nerve entrapment, fracture)

prevention and treatment of secondary effects of disuse and guarding (e.g., contractures, atrophy, weakness, edema)

interruption of nociception, pain, and underlying physiologic causes

prevention and treatment of the associated suffering, pain behaviors, disability, and psychological reaction.

This article focuses on the pharmacologic and physical medicine treatments, recognizing that a multidisciplinary or interdisciplinary approach including psychological and vocational counseling is often necessary.

From The Medical Center, Beaver, Pennsylvania (MCB); and the Department of Physical Medicine and Rehabilitation, Michigan State University, East Lansing, Michigan (MTA)

PHYSICAL MEDICINE AND REHABILITATION CLINICS OF NORTH AMERICA

Reports of the natural history of RSD and related problems is unknown and variable, depending on the author. Some reports suggest that the problem is self-limiting, but other authors report cases of long-term problems that last many years. Most reports of treatment are anecdotal; thus, confidently making treatment decisions is very difficult. A wide variety of treatments have been proposed, including conservative therapy, physical therapy, numerous regional blocks, systemic medications, transcutaneous nerve stimulation (TNS), surgical sympathectomy, cryotherapy, psychological counseling, and others.[7, 16]

TREATMENT OF THE PRECIPITATING CAUSE

If there is an identifiable inciting medical condition contributing to or causing RSD, such as nerve entrapment, adhesive capsulitis, or fracture, it is imperative to attempt to treat it as one of the first steps, e.g., it is appropriate to pursue surgical treatment for carpal tunnel syndrome if this is the presumed cause of the RSD.

PREVENTION OR REVERSAL OF DISUSE SEQUELAE

The pain caused by RSD often causes the patient to stop using his or her limb and thus leads to secondary consequences from disuse. These problems include contracture affecting the muscle, tendon, or joint; muscle atrophy; weakness; edema; and osteoporosis. These secondary complications can then take on an identity of their own and become a secondary or even the primary cause of pain and disability. Indeed, the disuse itself may be the inciting event that causes RSD, e.g., a fracture is placed in a cast and immobilized, and RSD symptoms then occur. Once these secondary complications have occurred, it becomes more difficult to differentiate the pain of RSD from the pain of disuse and stretching of contractures. The primary treatment of RSD must include the prevention and treatment of sequelae from guarding and protecting an extremity.

The reasons why people stop moving their extremity in RSD are very complex. The major reason seems to be the pain and pain tolerance, but other problems, including paralysis and psychosocial, vocational, family, legal, and medical issues, also strongly influence the patient's behavior and must be considered in the treatment program. Usually, the most important part of treatment in RSD is increasing or maintaining activities, and all strategies of treatment should be employed to achieve this goal. In addition to preventing the secondary effects of disuse, active exercise may theoretically normalize the underlying abnormal neurophysiology of RSD, thus decreasing pain. Blocks or medications should be followed immediately with specific therapeutic programs, usually in physical or occupational therapy.

Treatment recommendations in the early stages of RSD should include as many normal functional activities as possible. The patient should be encouraged to work, to dress himself or herself, and to use his or her extremity in the most normal way possible even though it hurts. Many cases of early RSD improve with simple activity and never require further intervention.

Patients who present with guarding and do not readily use their limb present a much more difficult set of problems. In these patients, the full spectrum of modalities and treatment options needs to be considered. Some authors advocate blocks, whereas others suggest systemic drug therapy, but nearly all authors advocate physical therapy in addition to any other modality.[7, 16, 23] Because there does not seem to be clear scientific evidence to favor one treatment over another, we suggest that each case be viewed individually, with the pros and cons of each therapy carefully considered before a treatment plan is outlined, e.g., we do not think it appropriate that a particular block be recommended to each patient without considering other treatments.

There have been no systematic and controlled studies evaluating specific exercise programs in RSD, but there are many different treatment options available. The treatment prescription for physical therapy and occupational therapy should include an active exercise program to involve all the joints and muscles of the limb. Active exercise can mobilize fluid; decrease edema; activate large nerve fiber proprioceptors (theoretically to lower pain perception, using the gate theory); improve muscle strength; increase range of motion (ROM); and desensitize the extremity. Some patients benefit from activity in the less affected joints earlier in the therapy session and save the most painful joint movement for the end. Additionally, a general aerobic exercise program to prevent further deconditioning and maximize the systemic benefits of exercise should be instituted.

Active exercise and ROM programs can be supplemented with passive ROM exercises and passive stretch, which can decrease contracture and improve overall limb function. Passive modalities can be useful temporarily to decrease pain and to increase activity. Transcutaneous electrical nerve stimulation (TENS), heat, or cold can assist with this goal. If a limb has already developed edema, then Jobst pumping, finger wrapping, or other pressure devices can control edema, which may translate into improved ROM. Contrast baths (alternating hot and cold exposure) may desensitize the limb[9] and also can be somewhat active in that the patient moves their limb to and from the different baths. It is not always necessary to precede the active physical therapy program with analgesics or nerve blocks, but in given patients these periods of decreased nociception and pain may allow the patient to increase their activity enough so that in their next therapy visit there is a noticeable gain.

Rarely is any surgical correction for contracture from RSD indicated. An occasional case could benefit from surgery to release a contracture or spasticity, but each case would need to be considered individually.

Often, behavioral treatment plans are necessary for treatment improvements in therapy. Operant programs should set specific, attainable goals, with continued treatment, medications, blocks, or modalities contingent on progress in therapy, e.g., a hot pack or medication can be used as a reinforcer after there have been measurable gains in therapy. Lack of progress in therapy can suggest the need for and justify changes in other portions or contingencies of the rehabilitation program.

SYSTEMIC PHARMACOTHERAPY

The relief of nociception or pain from RSD may not be solely dependent on interruption of sympathetic activity; rather, relief may in part be attributable to vasodilation and increased peripheral blood flow. Nitroglycerin and calcium channel blockers produce vasodilation without specific sympatholytic effects. The use of nitroglycerin in the treatment of RSD is described in a case report in which a patient treated for angina pectoris noted decreased swelling, stiffness, and pain associated with his chronic hand pain. Symptoms recurred on discontinuation of use of the transcutaneous nitroglycerin disks but remitted again when therapy was reinstituted.[21] Therapy with oral nifedipine was initiated in 13 patients with RSD in an open-label trial. Doses ranged from 10 to 30 mg three times daily and were tapered over several days after the patient had achieved a "stable level of pain relief" for 3 weeks. If pain recurred, therapy was reinstituted. Seven patients reported complete pain relief, 2 had partial relief, 3 withdrew because of side effects, and 1 patient failed to achieve adequate pain relief.[25]

α-Adrenergic antagonists selectively block the effects of epinephrine and norepinephrine and may produce improvement in patients with RSD. Phenoxybenzamine was dispensed to 40 consecutive patients with causalgia within 4 weeks of the onset of pain. Total resolution of pain was achieved in all cases after 6 to 8 weeks of therapy using doses of 40 to 120 mg per day. Side effects included orthostatic hypotension and reduction of seminal fluid (the authors cited "ejaculatory problems") but did not result in an interruption of therapy.[14] Prazosin, a selective competitive inhibitor of α_1-adrenergic receptors, has also been recommended to relieve symptoms of RSD.[30]

Propranolol, presumably by decreasing sympathetic outflow from the central nervous system, has also been recommended for relief of RSD. Therapy was maintained in two patients for 3 months at a dosage of 240 mg/d and subsequently discontinued without relapse of symptoms.[29]

The efficacy of oral corticosteroid therapy is notable in that duration of symptoms did not influence response to treatment. A prospective study (without a control group) of 64 patients with symptoms of RSD suggests that as many as 82% of patients experience at least a 50% reduction in their symptoms. Patients received oral prednisone, starting at a dosage of 60 to 80 mg daily and then gradually tapered over a 3- to 4-week period.[23]

A prospective randomized double-blind study using intranasal salmon calcitonin to treat RSD has recently been reported. Thirty-three patients in each group received either calcitonin or placebo, in combination with a physical treatment and physiotherapy program. Pain, ROM, edema, ability to work, and adverse reactions were measured. The calcitonin group showed significantly better improvement characterized by decreased pain at rest and on movement. A trend was also noted toward enhanced ability to work in the calcitonin group.[16] Another trial, in which physical therapy was not used, did not show a benefit for intranasal calcitonin.[4] Intranasal calcitonin, however, is not generally available in the United States.

Although personal experience suggests that opioids have limited effectiveness in most patients with RSD, especially those with long-standing pain, the use of opioids early in treatment may provide sufficient symptomatic relief to augment rehabilitation by improving the patient's acceptance of passive and active physical modalities.

Heterocyclic antidepressant medications are frequently used in treating patients with chronic pain. Their effectiveness is not dependent on the presence of clinical depression, and their use in a variety of chronic pain disorders has been described.[7] Although its mechanism of action is not fully understood with respect to pain relief, the benefits of antidepressant therapy may at least be partially attributed to an improvement in sleep patterns in chronic pain patients. Clinical use is occasionally limited by intolerable anticholinergic side effects.

Membrane-stabilizing agents such as phenytoin and carbamazepine are used clinically for patients experiencing neuropathic pain such as trigeminal neuralgia. Although sympathetic hyperactivity is often associated with neural trauma and neuropathic pain, the utility of membrane stabilizers in relieving nonlancinating pain is suspect.

SELECTIVE SYMPATHETIC GANGLION BLOCKADE

Alleviation of pain from selective sympathetic blockade has been advocated as the standard to confirm the diagnosis of RSD. In addition to diagnostic utility, selective sympathetic blockade using local anesthetics has evolved into a mainstay of therapy for RSD. Bonica et al[7] suggest that sympathetic blockade in combination with vigorous physical therapy "cures" approximately 80% of patients with RSD.

Pain relief often outlasts the pharmacologic effects of the local anesthetic. This observation is frequently described as "breaking the cycle" of nociceptor sensitization by sympathetic overactivity. Occasionally, these techniques are limited in their usefulness, by providing relief that does not last beyond the few hours of pharmacologic effectiveness of the local anesthetic. When this is the case, temporary relief may still be of benefit by enhancing the patient's tolerance of concurrent therapy (e.g., physical therapy). In contrast to somatic nerve blocks, such as epidural or brachial plexus nerve blocks, selective sympathetic nerve blocks do not interrupt motor or somatosensory nerve function. The patient therefore experiences pain relief without functional impairment of the extremity, allowing him or her to participate in active physical therapy modalities.

Reflex sympathetic dystrophy of the head, neck, or upper extremities can be relieved by injection of local anesthetic solution at the cervicothoracic ganglion (stellate ganglion). Failure to achieve complete sympathetic interruption of the upper extremity by direct stellate ganglion blockade may occasionally be due to anatomical variation. Kuntz's nerve's, anomalous pathways from the second and third thoracic nerves, bypass the stellate ganglion and enter the brachial plexus via the first thoracic nerve.[6] Alternative approaches to accomplish sympathetic interruption into the upper extremity, although not sympathetically selective, include brachial plexus blockade and interpleural injection of local anesthetic.[10, 26]

Complications associated with stellate ganglion blockade include central nervous system depression or excitation, including seizures due to local anesthetic toxicity (direct vertebral artery injection); high-level neural blockade and respiratory arrest from inadvertent subarachnoid injection; pneumothorax; recurrent laryngeal nerve blockade, with corresponding hoarseness and compromised ability to protect the airway; phrenic nerve blockade; neuritis; osteitis; and hematoma.[8] The appearance of Horner's syndrome (ptosis, myosis, enophthalmos, and anhidrosis) is expected, as are nasal congestion and conjunctival injection, serving as evidence of sympathetic blockade but not necessarily indicative of complete sympathetic interruption of the upper extremity. Temperature increase in the ipsilateral extremity is also expected.

The lumbar sympathetic chain lies on the anterolateral vertebral column, providing sympathetic innervation to the pelvic viscera and lower extremities. Selective sympathetic blockade is classically accomplished by injecting solution at the L2, L3, and L4 levels, necessitating three separate injection sites. Alternatively, a single injection site at approximately the L3 vertebral body may produce blockade of the lumbar sympathetic chain by using a larger volume (10–15 mL) of injectate that spreads cephalad and caudad within the prevertebral fascial plane.[19] Complications associated with lumbar sympathetic nerve blocks include aortic or inferior vena caval puncture, renal perforation, neuritis, osteitis, hypotension, and subarachnoid injection.

A variety of local anesthetic agents have been used for sympathetic blockade. Clinical preference of an agent is commonly based on the duration of desired pharmacologic effect and associated side effects. Empiric evidence defining the optimal interval between repeated injections is lacking; however, clinical practice suggests that aggressive, early therapy yields the best results. A schedule of daily or every-other-day injections is frequently prescribed for as long as the pain continues to improve or until complete relief is achieved. Continuous local anesthetic infusions using percutaneous catheters can be used in an inpatient setting.

The administration of regional anesthetic techniques is generally labor- or resource-intensive, or both. Anatomically precise administration of local anesthetic requires a specialist working in a theater equipped with resuscitation equipment. Many practices use routine blood pressure and electrocardiographic monitoring during and after each procedure. Patients are often instructed to avoid oral intake to reduce the risk of regurgitation and aspiration. Intravenous access is established prior to the procedure to allow rapid administration of emergency drugs when needed. Anticoagulation, local infection, and sepsis are contraindications to invasive regional anesthetic techniques.

NEUROLYTIC TECHNIQUES

When local anesthetic therapy is limited by a short duration of pain relief without progressive improvement, neurolytic agents such as 6% phenol or 50% alcohol can be administered in similar fashion. Because of the relatively nonreversible nature of these agents and potentially catastrophic consequences of misapplied solutions, radiographic guidance (e.g., with fluoroscopy) is recommended to document the location of the needle tip prior to injection. Initial injection of local anesthetic solution immediately prior to the application of the neurolytic agent serves as a test dose and may decrease the discomfort associated with alcohol or phenol injection. The use of contrast media to document the spread of solution through the fascial plane has also been recommended to reduce the risk of untoward complications.

Neurolytic sympathectomy can also be performed surgically or by radiofrequency denervation. These techniques are especially useful for cervical sympathectomy, because of the proximity of the roots of the brachial plexus. The risk of inadvertent somatic nerve injury and postsympathectomy neuralgia may be reduced when compared with chemical neurolysis.[20] The comparative efficacy of chemical, surgical, and radiofrequency neurolysis in accomplishing long-term pain relief is unknown. In an extensive review of the literature, most authors report that complete relief of burning pain from causalgia is achieved in more than 85% of patients after preganglionic sympathectomy.[7] Similar results are also suggested in relieving the pain associated with RSD. Failure in providing complete pain relief is generally attributed to incomplete sympathetic denervation or poor patient selection. The patient's tolerance of side effects and complications such as persistent Horner's syndrome (cervical) or impotence (lumbar) must be considered before an irreversible lesion is created. The potential for recurrent pain or debilitating deafferentation pain in long-term follow-up may also limit the utility of a neurodestructive approach.

INTRAVENOUS REGIONAL SYMPATHETIC BLOCKADE

Intravenous regional nerve blocks, frequently termed Bier blocks, are performed by isolating the patient's limb with a pneumatic tourniquet. After intravenous access is established, using a small catheter in the distal extremity, the limb is exsanguinated with an Esmarch wrap and the tourniquet is inflated. Typically, a tourniquet pressure of 50 mm Hg above systolic blood pressure is recommended for the arm, and 100 mm Hg above systolic blood pressure, for the leg. The injectate is administered by the intravenous catheter, and the tourniquet remains inflated 10 to 30 minutes allowing for fixation of the drug to local tissues. The tourniquet is deflated slowly to minimize peak systemic drug levels and to allow observation of signs or symptoms of drug toxicity.

Intravenous access may be difficult to establish in patients with vasoconstriction due to RSD. Access can often be facilitated by topical application of nitroglycerin ointment.[11] Performance of a stellate ganglion nerve block or lumbar epidural nerve block can be used to produce vasodilation for intravenous access and to improve the tolerance of a patient's hyperesthetic limb to the tight wrapping of an elastic Esmarch bandage.[13]

Hannington-Kiff is credited with first describing the use of intravenous regional sympathetic blockade, using guanethidine for RSDs of the limbs. Since that time the efficacy of reserpine,[3] bretylium,[12] ketanserin,[17] and ketorolac[31] has been described for similar use.

Guanethidine, 10 to 20 mg, is diluted in 25 to 50 mL isotonic saline for injection into the arm or leg respectively.[18] Bretylium, 1 to 3 mg/kg, is shorter acting than guanethidine, and its use may need to be repeated more frequently. Heparin, 500 to 1000 IU, is often added to the solution to reduce the risk of intravascular coagulation. Local anesthetics can be used in lieu of isotonic saline to decrease tourniquet pain and the discomfort of injection secondary to norepinephrine release.

Guanethidine is a "false transmitter," accumulating and displacing norepinephrine from intraneuronal storage granules in nerve terminals. Restoration of norepinephrine stores is dependent on axonal transport of new storage vesicles, which takes 5 to 7 weeks in animal studies. Bretylium does not deplete norepinephrine stores acutely; rather, it inhibits the release of norepinephrine when the nerve terminal is depolarized. Long-term use however, does result in norepinephrine depletion. Reserpine antagonizes the uptake of norepinephrine by inhibiting the ATP-Mg++ dependent mechanism of the chromaffin granule membrane.[15] Guanethidine and injectable reserpine are generally unavailable in the United States, limiting the clinical use of Bier blocks in the treatment of RSD.

The most frequent side effects associated with guanethidine, reserpine, and bretylium are hypotension, flushing, lightheadedness, and syncope. Reserpine, a tertiary amine, is associated with a higher incidence of central nervous system effects, including sedation and a state of indifference to environmental stimuli, because of its ability to easily cross the blood–brain barrier. Bretylium, a quaternary ammonium compound, and guanethidine, a strongly basic moiety, have few central nervous system effects.

Phentolamine has been administered intravenously as a diagnostic tool and prognostic indicator of responsiveness to intravenous regional guanethidine therapy. Phentolamine has a relatively transient albeit more rapid onset of α blockade when compared with phenoxybenzamine. Patients receive 5 to 15 mg of intravenous phentolamine over a 5- to 10-minute period. All of the 53 patients who experienced relief of ongoing and evoked pain with phentolamine subsequently reported pain relief after regional guanethidine.[1]

A randomized trial of 19 patients showed no difference in therapeutic efficacy in 1-month and 3-month follow-up comparing stellate ganglion blocks every day, to a total of 8 blocks, and intravenous regional guanethidine every 4 days, to a total of 4 blocks. The intravenous guanethidine group also showed persistent increases in skin temperature and plethysmographic waves at 24 and 48 hours after injection, compared with the stellate ganglion block group.[5]

Similar to other regional anesthetic techniques, intravenous regional blocks require rigorous patient monitoring and immediate availability of resuscitation equipment.

ELECTROSTIMULATION

An uncontrolled study of TENS produced good-to-excellent pain relief in 20 of 29 patients (mean age 43 years) with the diagnosis of RSD.[27] In a separate study, 7 of 10 children had complete remission of symptoms within 2 months of initiation of TENS and physical therapy.[22] A study of seven healthy volunteers demonstrated increased infrared emission (by thermogram) distal to the site of electric stimulation and elevations in cutaneous temperatures. The investigators postulated that these results indicated cutaneous vasodilation and decreased sympathetic tone.[24] Unfortunately, many patients do not tolerate TENS because of increased pain.

Epidural spinal cord stimulation produced good or excellent results in 7 of 8 patients, with a follow-up of 27 months. A close relation between pain relief and increased peripheral blood flow, evidenced by thermography and plethysmography, was noted. Morbidity included local infection in 1 patient and electrode displacement in 2 patients.[27] Barolat and Ketcik[2] reported a series of 90 patients treated with epidural spinal cord stimulation in whom other forms of "aggressive" management had failed. Half the patients reported "some" pain relief (between 20% and 40%), and one third of the systems were removed because of lack of efficacy.

Although experience is limited, electrostimulation appears to offer some advantage to patients with intractable pain unremitting to alternative forms of therapy.

MULTIDIMENSIONAL ASPECTS OF PAIN

As with any patient suffering from chronic pain, assessment must include an evaluation of the patient's biomedical, psychosocial and behavioral condition to formulate a comprehensive treatment strategy. Evaluation and treatment by an integrated team of physical therapists, occupational therapists, psychologists, vocational rehabilitation counselors, nutritionists, social workers, nurses, physicians, and others are often necessary to address the entangled myriad of problems faced by patients with chronic pain. Patients must also be enlisted to become active participants in their treatment plan.

Simplistic approaches using isolated modalities (e.g., pharmacotherapy, surgical intervention) are often insufficient to return the patient to a satisfying and productive lifestyle. Focus must not be directed solely at the painful extremity; rather, therapy must include amelioration of concurrent symptoms of sleep disturbance, affective distress, marital discord, vocational disability, and any other maladaptive process associated with the patient's painful condition.

CONCLUSION

There are many different treatments available for RSD. Treatment of the precipitating cause and then increasing physical activity are the cornerstones of therapy. Regional blocks, systemic medications, or electrostimulation in combination with therapy offers the most common modalities for primary initial treatment. The earlier treatment is instituted, the better the response. Nonphysical, psychological, and vocational factors need to be considered in every patient, and multidisciplinary and interdisciplinary team treatment may be necessary.

References

1. Arnér S: Intravenous phentolamine test: Diagnostic and prognostic use in reflex sympathetic dystrophy. Pain 46:17–22, 1991
2. Barolat G, Ketcik B: Epidural spinal cord stimulation in the management of chronic pain in reflex sympathetic dystrophy. American Pain Society Abstract 91244, 1991
3. Benzon HT, Chomka CM, Brunner EA: Treatment of reflex sympathetic dystrophy with regional intravenous reserpine. Anesth Analg 59:500–502, 1980
4. Bickerstaff DR, Kanis JA: The use of nasal calcitonin in the treatment of post-traumatic algodystrophy. Br J Rheumatol 30:291–294, 1991
5. Bonelli S, Conoscente F, Movilia PG, et al: Regional intravenous guanethidine vs. stellate ganglion block in reflex sympathetic dystrophies: A randomized trial. Pain 16:297–307, 1983
6. Bonica JJ: Sympathetic Nerve Blocks for Pain Diagnosis and Therapy, volume II. Technical Considerations. New York, Breon Laboratories, 1981, p 66
7. Bonica JJ, Loeser JD, Chapman CR, et al: The Management of Pain, volume I, Ed 2. Philadelphia, Lea & Febiger, 1990, pp 220–243
8. Cousins MJ, Bridenbaugh PO: Neural Blockade in Clinical Anesthesia and Management of Pain. Philadelphia, Lippincott, 1988
9. DeLisa JA, Currie DM, Gans BM, et al: Rehabilitation Medicine: Principles and Practice. Philadelphia, JB Lippincott, 1988, p 260
10. Durrani Z, Winnie AP: Diagnostic and therapeutic brachial plexus block for RSD unresponsive to stellate ganglion block. Anesth Analg 74:S77, 1992
11. Foley K, Schatz L: Topical nitroglycerin facilitates intravenous regional techniques in patients with reflex sympathetic dystrophy. Anesthesiology 69:1029, 1988
12. Ford SR, Forrest WH, Etherington L: The treatment of reflex sympathetic dystrophy with intravenous regional bretylium. Anesthesiology 68:137–140, 1988
13. Gargiulo RF: A method of facilitating intravenous regional bretylium. Anesthesiology 69:147, 1988
14. Ghostine SY, Comair YG, Turner DM, et al: Phenoxybenzamine in the treatment of causalgia. J Neurosurg 60:1263–1268, 1984
15. Gilman AG, Rall TW, Nies AS, et al: Goodman and Gilman's The Pharmacological Basis of Therapeutics. New York, Pergamon Press, 1990
16. Gobelet C, Waldburger M, Meier JL: The effect of adding calcitonin to physical treatment of reflex sympathetic dystrophy. Pain 48:171–175, 1992
17. Hanna MH, Peat SJ: Ketanserin in reflex sympathetic dystrophy: A double-blind placebo controlled cross-over trial. Pain 38:145–150, 1989
18. Hannington-Kiff JG: Intravenous regional sympathetic block with guanethidine. Lancet 1019–1020, 1974
19. Hatangdi VS, Boas RA: Lumbar sympathectomy: A single needle technique. Br J Anaesth 57:285–289, 1985
20. Haynsworth RF, Noe CE: Percutaneous lumbar sympathectomy: A comparison of radiofrequency denervation versus phenol neurolysis. Anesthesiology 74:459–463, 1991
21. Hyland WT: Treating reflex sympathetic dystrophy with transdermal nitroglycerin. Plast Reconstr Surg 83:195, 1989
22. Kesler RW, Saulsbury FT, Miller LT, et al: Reflex sympathetic dystrophy in children: Treatment with transcutaneous electric nerve stimulation. Pediatrics 82:728–732, 1988
23. Kozin F, Ryan LM, Carrera GF, et al: The reflex sympathetic dystrophy syndrome (RSDS). III. Scintigraphic studies: Further evidence for the therapeutic efficacy of systemic corticosteroids and proposed diagnostic criteria. Am J Med 70:23–29, 1981
24. Owens S, Atkinson ER, Lees DE: Thermographic evidence of reduced sympathetic tone with transcutaneous nerve stimulation. Anesthesiology 50:62–65, 1979

25. Prough DS, McLeskey CH, Poehling GG, et al: Efficacy of oral nifedipine in the treatment of reflex sympathetic dystrophy. Anesthesiology 62:796–799, 1985
26. Reiestad F, McIlvaine WB, et al: Interpleural analgesia in treatment of upper extremity reflex sympathetic dystrophy. Anesth Analg 69:671–673, 1989
27. Robaina FJ, Dominguez M, et al: Spinal cord stimulation for relief of chronic pain in vasospastic disorders of the upper limbs. Neurosurgery 24:63–67, 1989
28. Robaina FJ, Rodriguez JL, de Vera JA, et al: Transcutaneous electrical nerve stimulation and spinal cord stimulation for pain relief in reflex sympathetic dystrophy. Sterotact Funct Neurosurg 52:53–62, 1989
29. Simson G: Propranolol for causalgia and sudek atrophy. JAMA 227:327, 1974
30. Spittell JA: Vasospastic disorders. Cardiovasc Clin 13(2):75–88, 1983
31. Vanos DN, Ramamurthy S, Hoffman J: Intravenous regional block using ketorolac: Preliminary results in the treatment of reflex sympathetic dystrophy. Anesth Analg 74:139–141, 1992

Address reprint requests to

Michael C. Brody, MD
2120 William Penn Highway
Pittsburgh, PA 15221

MODERN MEDICAL ELECTRICITY IN THE MANAGEMENT OF PAIN

C. Norman Shealy, MD, PhD, and Charles C. Mauldin, Jr, MD

Electrotherapy for pain management has experienced tremendous growth in the past 15 years.[9] The publication of the gate control theory by Melzack and Wall in 1965 seems to have been responsible for the proliferation of electric devices. Conventional transcutaneous electric nerve stimulation (TENS) was the first such device to be studied and used clinically. Various other transcutaneous devices have evolved and are differentiated from conventional TENS by their differing stimulus parameters. These include microcurrent, high- and low-voltage therapies, interferential stimulation, and cranial electrical stimulation. Percutaneous techniques include percutaneous electrical nerve stimulation and spinal cord stimulation. Deep brain stimulation is not discussed here. Iontophoresis is included as an electric therapy because current is required to drive ions through the skin. The therapeutic indications (Table 1) and contraindications of each of these techniques are discussed in this article. Most have little research to support their claims of benefit.

Acknowledgment of the history of electrotherapy may help us to maintain an appropriately skeptical perspective when we are called on to endorse the latest device by someone who believes in it. The roots of the specialty of physical medicine and rehabilitation can be traced to the rather bizarre practice (by today's standards) of electrotherapeutics from the seventeenth century into the twentieth century.[13] Outside the mainstream of medical practice, these physicians later expanded their "cures" to include other physical medicine modalities. Electrotherapy was touted to cure gynecologic conditions, hysteria, depression, paralysis, and other problems. Interest in electrotherapeutics declined when the American Medical Association denied affiliation in the early twentieth century. Krusen[15] states: "One dislikes to discuss charlatans, but physical medicine, because of its very nature, has had more than its share of irregular practitioners." On a positive note, Duchenne, credited as the founder of modern medical electrotherapeutics, did discover that faradic current could cause muscle contraction. Robert Remak built on this knowledge, accurately determining motor points.[15]

From Shealy Institute (CNS) and Cox Medical Centers (CCM), Springfield, Missouri

PHYSICAL MEDICINE AND REHABILITATION CLINICS
OF NORTH AMERICA

Table 1. INDICATIONS FOR ELECTRIC MODALITIES

	TENS	AL-TENS	PENS	IFT	HVS	LV-MS	PEMT	CES
Acute pain	***	****	***		**	*		
Chronic pain	****	****	***	*		*		**
Postoperative pain	**	***	**					
Joint pain	**	**	*	***				
Soft tissue injury	**	**	*		**	**	**	
Low back pain	****	**	***					**
Neck pain	***		**				**	**
Tendinitis	**			***			*	
Headache	**		**					**

Modalities are rated by supporting research or general acceptance. No stars indicates little or no support; four stars indicates a large body of supporting data and wide acceptance. TENS = Transcutaneous electric nerve stimulation; AL-TENS = Acupuncturelike TENS; PENS = percutaneous electrical nerve stimulation; IFT = interferential current therapy; HVS = high-voltage stimulation; LV-MS = low-voltage microampere stimulation; PEMT = pulsed electromagnetic therapy; CES = cranial electric stimulation.

The placebo effect should also be kept in mind when electrical therapies are used. A competent therapist who touches the patient and has any type of machine has at least a 30% chance of cure. Basmajian[1] states: "Only a naive person believes that nonspecific effects do not play an important part in the treatment of disabilities met with in a rehabilitation clinic, even in the treatment of patients with severe physical handicaps. The placebo response is not confined to patients with the usual types of psychosomatic ailments. It is found throughout all physical medicine, and it often is the most significant element in the treatment of patients with severe musculoskeletal problems." Nonspecific effects of therapy may be reasonable to use, provided that the risk of harm, both physical and financial, is low. Placebo electrotherapy is usually preferable to placebo surgery. We must, as medical scientists, seek to separate specific from nonspecific effects of treatment, realizing that our most beloved therapy may ultimately be shown to have no specific benefit.

TRANSCUTANEOUS ELECTRICAL NERVE STIMULATION

TENS is the best known, most widely used, and best-researched electric modality available today. More than 600 publications support its efficacy. Proponents of TENS include C. Norman Shealy,[29] Joel DeLisa,[7] Frederic Kottke,[14] Mathew Lee,[17] Jeffrey Saal,[28] and John Bonica,[4] to mention only a few. Despite the epidemiological study by Richard Deyo and co-workers[8] refuting the effectiveness of TENS, this technology continues to be widely used and reimbursed. The study by Deyo et al has been criticized from several points of view. Electrodes were placed only over the area of pain. The level of stimulation may have been too low and was not individualized. TENS was used for relatively short periods: 45 minutes. There was no mention of using acupuncturelike stimulation. Three more recent articles provide a much better perspective on TENS.[10, 40, 41]

History

In late 1967, Shealy began using the Electreat, a transcutaneous electrical nerve stimulator, to demonstrate to patients the feeling to be expected from dorsal column stimulation. He found that many patients achieved adequate pain relief with this device. This early TENS was found to give effective pain relief in the majority of chronic pain patients that Shealy was seeing. By 1971, he was inserting dorsal column stimulators in only 6% of chronic pain patients. He then developed a multimodal, multidisciplinary program emphasizing TENS, percutaneous electrical nerve stimulation (PENS), physical exercise, and behavioral techniques. Later, solid-state TENS devices became available, each with a characteristic frequency or wave form, or both. More recent advances have involved random or burst stimulus output, designed to prevent sensory accommodation. Many different TENS electrodes are now available, each modifying stimulation at least as much as does the TENS itself.

Of all the electrical modalities, TENS is by far the most widely used, even though its use is considerably less than desirable. In the Nuprin Pain Report, less than 2% of individuals reported being offered a TENS device for back pain, despite numerous reports of an efficacy rate of 80% in most acute low back pain problems and of at least 50% in most chronic low back pain problems. Pomeranz[26] cites a number of controlled clinical studies that have shown that TENS outperforms sham TENS. Wolfe et al[44] report that TENS is effective in 60% of acute pain of any source and 75% of patients with chronic, intractable pain, which is often refractory to conventional methods. TENS should be considered as the primary treatment choice for virtually any type of pain. Shealy has shown that a combination of TENS and use of a guided imagery–relaxation audio tape leads to a 50% to 100% pain reduction in 80% of chronic pain patients. The Food and Drug Administration's report on TENS concluded that TENS is a safe, effective pain therapy when used by a person with adequate medical knowledge and training in the method.[23] The report of the Office of Inspector General of the US Department of Health and Human Services in 1990 reports that 80% of the people receiving TENS benefited. The conclusion was that the Health Care Financing Administration should reimburse providers of TENS.[42]

Advantages of TENS

TENS is virtually totally safe. The side effects of drugs can often be avoided with use of TENS. The long-term cost of treatment may be less with TENS than with medication, and it may be safer than even over-the-counter pain medications.

Side Effects

Approximately 1.5% of patients have cutaneous sensitivity or allergy to the electrode gel. This problem is greatly reduced by the use of karaya self-adherent pads. Other measures to control skin irritation include moving the electrodes, cleaning the electrodes, and using corticosteroid creams. Skin irritation has also been reported to be caused by electric effects. This is minimized by using biphasic pulses (with zero-net direct current) and placement of electrodes to avoid "hot spots" of high-current density.[11]

Application of TENS

Application is the most crucial part of TENS therapy. Poor placement or application is the most common reason for TENS failure. In general, "search" electrodes should be placed on either side of the painful area or above and below the site of pain. Rarely is TENS most efficacious directly over the area of the pain, and direct application is particularly unwise in acute pain. Once the electrodes are placed, the patient is asked to increase the amplitude of each channel (usually two) of the TENS device slowly to a level that is slightly uncomfortable. Then, the intensity should be adjusted to a point just below the discomfort level.

Most patients prefer a relatively rapid pulse rate, so it is advisable to begin with maximal frequency and then suggest that they compare the lowest, medium, and highest frequencies. Most TENS devices today offer modulation such as on-off burst, automatic frequency, and intensity adjustments. Some devices offer a pre-programmed pattern of varying frequency and intensity so that virtually no accommodation occurs. Other devices also overcome habituation by delivering random stimuli. Godfrey[11] refers to this feature as *antihabituation.*

When patients do not achieve a reduction of pain of 50% or more within 30 to 60 minutes, the electrode positions should be altered to ensure that electric paresthesia is occurring in the area of pain. If paresthesia is occurring but is inadequate for pain control, the frequency should be adjusted to the lowest setting and the amplitude increased to as high a level as tolerated. Once pain relief is adequate (75% or greater), the device should be worn continuously from morning until bedtime. The patient should remove electrodes on the first evening to assess skin tolerance. Some electrodes may be left in place for 2 or 3 days if there has been no skin irritation. Electrode wires simply need to be disconnected for bathing. In extensive experience with 8000 patients at the Shealy Institute, low-amplitude current is rarely effective with short applications, and continuous use during the day is indicated. After a few weeks, patients may obtain satisfactory relief using TENS on an as-needed basis. With chronic pain, about 50% of patients need the TENS and retraining cassette tapes for only 3 to 6 months. Most of the others require long-term TENS use, for as much as decades.

Conventional TENS (Sensory-Level TENS, Low-Intensity TENS)

Large-diameter afferents are thought to be stimulated at low intensity and to reduce the sensation of pain by the gate theory. The current used should not exceed a level twice the threshold for sensation. The frequency is considered high at 100 to 200 Hz, which is thought to maximize presynaptic inhibition mediated by γ-aminobutyric acid. The pulse duration ranges from 2 to 50 microseconds. Additional effects occur through descending inhibitory pathways from the midbrain, releasing monoamines (serotonin and epinephrine) in the spinal cord.[26]

Analgesia from conventional TENS starts within seconds of onset of stimulation and disappears soon after the stimulator is turned off. Naloxone does not block conventional TENS, indicating a mechanism of pain relief other than one that is endorphin mediated. This form of TENS is effective for acute and chronic pain, but perhaps it is best for acute pain.[37] It is effective in postoperative pain,[39] low back pain,[28] pancreatitis,[27] and postherpetic neuralgia.[19] It is well tolerated and is clearly the first choice in electrotherapy. Stimulus adaptation may preclude prolonged effectiveness. As mentioned earlier, more recent devices may be able to prevent this.

All patients sent home with TENS after the initial demonstration of effectiveness should be adequately instructed, both verbally and in writing, in the care and maintenance of the device, battery changing, and electrode placement. Shealy believes that a guided-imagery relaxation tape should also be provided for use at least four times a day for the first 2 weeks and twice a day thereafter. The patient should be seen at 2 to 4 weeks, earlier if pain relief is inadequate.

Acupuncturelike TENS (AL-TENS, Intense TENS, Motor-Level TENS, Noninvasive Electroacupuncture)

Acupuncturelike TENS uses low frequency (4 Hz) and a stimulus intensity sufficient to produce muscle contraction. The stimulation of muscle afferents is thought to release endorphins. Naloxone blocks AL-TENS. Additionally, the pituitary is thought to release adrenocorticotropic hormone along with endorphins, stimulating the adrenals to release cortisol. Acupuncture analgesia is characterized by a "de gi" sensation at the point of needle insertion. This same dull ache is produced by AL-TENS, perhaps explaining the logic for referring to this therapy as acupuncturelike.

A wide pulse width of 1000 microseconds is required. Conventional TENS devices are not capable of this pulse width. Frequency must be kept low, or painful tetany will occur.

Onset of pain relief is from 20 to 30 minutes and may last from hours to days. Daily treatment appears to have a cumulative effect. AL-TENS does not have to be placed in the area of pain to be effective and may work well over acupuncture or trigger points. Unfortunately, some patients do not tolerate stimulation strong enough to produce muscle contraction and therefore cannot benefit from this treatment modality. AL-TENS is most effective in chronic, deep, throbbing, or arthritic pain.

Noxious-Level TENS

When adjustments in electrodes, frequency, patterning, and intensity do not lead to satisfactory pain control, it is advisable in chronic pain to apply the electrodes directly over the area of pain. The amplitude should be increased to an intensity as strong as the patient tolerates for 20 minutes. Only the Electreat and Com-TENS are likely to be strong enough for this approach. If intense TENS gives pain relief, patients may be instructed to use it 20 minutes eight times a day for at least 2 weeks, often with satisfactory relief thereafter, using it only four times per day or less.

TENS Electrodes

For initial trials of TENS in the office, sponge electrodes are ideal because they require only water and are sterilizable and capable of prolonged reuse. They allow one to "search" without using the more expensive disposable electrodes. Once satisfactory electric paresthesia is achieved in the area of pain, the disposable, self-adhering electrodes should be provided. At the Shealy Institute, the following brands of electrodes have been found to be most useful and cost effective: NTRON Ntrode (NTRON, Sugar Land, TX); Empi Soft Touch (Empi, St. Paul, MN); and Medical Designs Progel (Medical Designs, St. Paul, MN). Surginet (Zens Health Care Products, Milwaukee, WI) or Coban (3M Healthcare, St. Paul, MN) also is very helpful to hold electrodes securely on extremities.

TENS Adjuncts

Shealy believes that at least 80% of chronic pain patients are deficient in magnesium and taurine, both essential nutrients and enhancers of electric energy. If patients do not respond to TENS or if it loses efficiency, a magnesium load test and an amino acid profile should be done. As deficiencies are corrected, the effectiveness of TENS may be greatly enhanced.[30, 34]

PERCUTANEOUS ELECTRICAL NERVE STIMULATION

Some 20 years ago, Shealy began using PENS,[32] inserting needles into the area of pain or near major peripheral nerves. The initial purpose was to demonstrate the sensation of electric nerve activation, although he found that some patients achieved excellent pain relief, occasionally lasting for days. Initially using 22-gauge spinal needles and, later, changing to solid needles of 28- to 32-gauge diameter, he demonstrated analgesia sufficient for surgical procedures such as laminectomy, craniotomy, and ulnar nerve transposition. This technique should be considered when TENS has been ineffective.

The needles are inserted above and below and into the central area of pain. Alligator clips are applied to the superior and inferior needles, and the amplitude is increased to a pleasant throb. A 5-Hz frequency with a pulse width of 0.5 milliseconds is used. If relief is not obtained within 15 minutes, the frequency may be decreased to 1 Hz, and the intensity to a level that is painful but tolerable for 20 minutes. The best stimulators are those sold for use by acupuncturists. Pain relief is often quite prolonged, as long as a week or more. If, by the third treatment (not done more often than three times a week), pain relief of several days is not achieved, regular PENS is unlikely to be helpful. As with TENS, it is crucial to obtain electric paresthesia in the area of pain. The needles may be adjusted to achieve this effect.

The depth of needle insertion depends on the body area treated. In the chest, the depth should be shallow enough to prevent the risk of pneumothorax. In the lumbar and cervical regions, needles are inserted deep enough to touch facets or transverse processes. For headache, the best location for PENS is with the positive leads over the C2 facets and the negative leads connected to a needle in the center of the first dorsal interosseous muscle of the ipsilateral hand. Additional needles placed to the lamina at T1 may sometimes be helpful.

Intense PENS

In a small but grateful group of patients, very intense PENS may offer excellent relief of pain. Shealy has found that the areas most amenable to this treatment are the sacroiliac joints and the paracoccygeal region (for pelvic or coccygeal pain). For sacroiliac joints, needles are inserted in the upper and lower aspects of the joint, unilaterally or bilaterally. In the paracoccygeal application, needles are placed on either side of the coccyx at a depth of approximately 1 cm.

Alligator clips are then attached to the needles either vertically, horizontally, or obliquely, depending on the elicited sensation. Shealy uses an early-model Stim-tech (Stimtech Corp., Minneapolis, MN), which has a higher output than any of the modern TENS devices. Pulse width and frequency are maximal. The patients are then asked to increase the amplitude slowly to a level that is just painful but tolerable. They are encouraged to continue adjusting intensity upward toward maximum every few minutes. The intense PENS is continued for 20 to 30 minutes. Analgesia and local anesthesia are often quite satisfactory and may exceed those of a local anesthetic. Effects may last hours or days. When effective, the treatment may be repeated as much as three times a week or as needed. If at least 1 week's improvement is not achieved after 6 treatments, use of intense PENS is discontinued. If the period of relief is increasing, as many as 15 treatments may be done initially, often with relief lasting up to many months. Occasional retreatment may be necessary. Shealy has noted occasional patients who achieve pain relief for years with repeated single treatments approximately three times per year.

DORSAL COLUMN STIMULATION

Many now refer to dorsal column stimulation (DCS) as *spinal cord stimulation*. Although Shealy no longer performs it and does not recommend implanted stimulators for pain control,[33, 36] many surgeons and anesthesiologists continue to recommend and implant these stimulators.[22] Law[16] provides a recent review of this technology for the failed back. Complications of this technique include paralysis, spinal cord injury, cerebrospinal fluid leaks, infection, failure of the stimulator, and fracture of the electrodes. Psychological counseling and adequate trials of TENS, PENS, and behavioral techniques should be undertaken prior to implantation of DCS. With an inadequate guarantee of long-term pain relief, DCS is unequivocally a procedure of last resort.

CRANIAL ELECTRIC STIMULATION

In 1975, Saul Liss introduced the Pain Suppressor and, later, the Liss CES (MediConsultants, Glen Rock, NJ) for relief of pain and anxiety, depression, and insomnia. Whether by cause or effect, the correlation between depression and chronic pain is clear. Shealy notes that 44% of patients having chronic pain have reported improvement when treated with cranial electric stimulation (CES). The Liss devices generate very high frequency stimulation, as much as 20,000 Hz in 15-Hz bursts. Shealy has shown a reversal of neurotransmitter imbalances associated with depression in 72% of patients treated for 20 minutes a day for 2 weeks.[31, 35]

When CES is used for headache, the electrodes should initially be placed suboccipitally. If pain relief is not achieved within 15 minutes, the following electrode combinations should be employed: nasion-inion, bitemporal, or frontal–occipital–first web space. In general, headache relief requires only 30 to 60 minutes of application and may be repeated as needed. Intensity should not exceed 2 mA, and 1 mA is often adequate. Patients should not experience a sense of electrical paresthesia with CES, because this may involve a current sufficient to create burns. At 0.5 to 1 mA, a visual flicker (similar to a fast strobe light) is induced so that patients are assured that they are achieving real treatment. When this device is applied, the intensity is slowly increased until the patient feels the sensation at the electrodes and then is reduced until the sensation disappears. The patient does not have to feel the current to derive benefit.

Further studies are needed to clarify usefulness of CES, but it appears to be safe for clinical use and has been demonstrated to alter β-endorphin and serotonin levels. It, like TENS, is contraindicated in patients with pacemakers and in pregnancy. Adverse effects have been limited to minor skin irritation from the electrodes.

INTERFERENTIAL CURRENT THERAPY

Interferential current therapy (IFT) was first introduced by Nemec in Vienna in 1950 and has been practiced sporadically throughout Europe ever since. IFT is more commonplace in rehabilitation practices in Europe than in North America. Current proponents of IFT in the United States include H.U. May, Francois Savery, and Robert G. Schwartz. Two alternating-current sine waves of differing frequencies produce an interferential current, also referred to as a *beat pulse* or *alternating modulation frequency*. Four electrodes are applied to the patient in such a way as to generate a beat pulse in the area of interest. Reportedly, this interferential current can stimulate sensory, motor, and pain fibers. Rather elaborate explanations of the therapeutic benefit have been confirmed by very little research. Claims have been made regarding the ability to selectively stimulate various tissue types by changing the available stimulus parameters. These parameters include pulse width, interpulse interval, frequency, current (or voltage), and wave-form configurations. Other variables may include the size, shape, and placement of electrodes and their impedance. The primary advantage of IFT appears to be that it is comfortable. Expense is a disadvantage.

The most common clinical use reported has been relief of pain in orthopedic conditions. IFT has also been proposed for edema control, stimulation of soft tissue healing, and other types of pain (reflex sympathetic dystrophy syndrome, peripheral vascular disease, ovarian cyst, diabetic neuropathy, and gangrene). Reasonably well documented relief has been shown in lateral epicondylitis, osteoarthritis of the knee, sprains, and jaw dysfunction. Patient comfort should dictate the intensity level used. Duration of treatment is 10 to 15 minutes, and 10 to 15 sessions should suffice for acute pain. Longer treatment may be needed in chronic disorders.

Contraindications

IFT should not be used in patients with tetany, inflammatory processes, bleeding disorders (especially if suction-cup applicators are used), or deep vein thrombosis or in patients with demand pacemakers. IFT is suspected to promote clotting through its effect on platelets.[20] Various manufacturers list precautions regarding skin disease, osteomyelitis, malignancy, seizure disorder, multiple sclerosis, and pregnancy. The stimulator should be kept at least 20 ft away from short-wave diathermy. The presence of a metallic prosthesis is not considered to be a contraindication, because there is no heat or current concentration.

HIGH-VOLTAGE STIMULATION

Bell Laboratories developed high-voltage stimulation (HVS) in the 1940s as a means of delivering current to deep tissues without damage to superficial tissues. This electric therapy is frequently, although incorrectly, referred to as *galvanic stimulation.* HVS provides a twin-peak, monophasic pulse of short duration (2 to 60 microseconds) and a high-peak current intensity (2000 to 2500 mA). A high driving voltage (as much as 500 V) is required to generate such a high peak current. This combination of parameters provides stimulation to sensory, motor, and pain fibers that is relatively comfortable and is popular for the treatment of pain. Although little research has been done, HVS appears sufficiently similar to other currents that produce electroanalgesia to allow its use in pain control. Sohn et al[38] demonstrated its usefulness in management of pain associated with levator ani syndrome. HVS has also been touted to accelerate wound healing. A multicenter study is currently under way to investigate this possibility. Contraindications are no different from those of TENS.

LOW-VOLTAGE MICROAMPERE STIMULATION

Low-voltage microampere stimulation (LV-MS, microcurrent) devices deliver a current of less than 1000 μA at 10 to 60 V. They are considered experimental when used for electroanalgesia. Picher[25] has been a proponent of this technique in the treatment of pain, inflammation, wound healing, and edema. Pape[24] has used this modality to improve motor function of nonspastic antagonist muscles in children with spastic diplegia. He also demonstrated improvement in muscle bulk and strength in patients with neurologic injuries. Carley and Wainapel[5] found that wounds healed 1.5 to 2.5 times faster with LV-MS than in matched controls. Precautions and contraindications are the same as for TENS.

PULSED ELECTROMAGNETIC THERAPY

Pain relief is a possible use of pulsed electromagnetic therapy (PEMT). Nolan et al[21] report a double-blind, crossover study of PEMT in cervical pain. All patients had persistent neck pain for longer than 8 weeks. With 3 weeks of therapy, 80% of patients reported that they were moderately better to much better. Visual analog pain scores dropped from 7 to 3. Cervical range of motion was improved and analgesic use had decreased significantly in the group receiving PEMT. Although the exact mechanism of action is unclear, a reduction in muscle spindle excitability from gamma fiber activation is proposed. Increased collagen extensibility with subsequent decreased joint stiffness and reduction in muscle spasm are also considerations. Several cellular enzymes have been found to be sensitive to PEMT.[18] Bassett et al[2] have demonstrated that PEMT shows a narrow therapeutic window in different tissues. The reduction in pain may be due to an anti-inflammatory or healing effect on any one of the number of tissues. Goldin et al[12] have reported increased rates of wound healing in patients receiving PEMT. Accelerated fracture healing has also been shown. Symptomatic pain relief has been reported to occur in patients with ankle sprains[43] and impingement syndrome.[3]

PEMT is applied daily for 2 to 8 hours. The magnetic fields generated may interfere with monitoring of electrocardiographic signals, as do other electric devices.

IONTOPHORESIS

Iontophoresis is a technique that uses galvanic current to drive charged particles into or through a biologic membrane. Because similarly charged particles are repelled, a positive ion is repelled from the anode, and vice versa. Weak solutions of drugs that are both water- and lipid-soluble may be iontophoresed. Corticosteroids, anesthetics, salicylates, and antibiotics have been used. At least one study[6] indicates that corticosteroids do not migrate through the skin. Studies reporting the benefit of iontophoresis of various drugs for a variety of musculoskeletal problems are inconclusive. It is likely that any drug that penetrates the skin is promptly delivered to the venous system through the subdermal plexus. Delivery of drug by injection or by mouth is preferred.

SUMMARY

With the economics of medical care and the history of electrotherapeutics firmly in mind, one should seek treatments that are efficient and effective. There is no question that relief of the symptom of pain must be a primary focus of treatment, whether or not a specific pathology is known. Electric devices may be justifiably used for their placebo effects, if the cost is reasonable, because side effects are minor and infrequent. Research shows specific neurochemical effects of several electrotherapeutic devices, supporting the notion that specific therapeutic effects exist in addition to placebo effects. Passage of time and further research will determine which of the current techniques and devices will find their way into future similar articles or monographs.

References

1. Basmajian JV: Biofeedback for neuromuscular rehabilitation. Critical Reviews in Physical Medicine and Rehabilitation 1:39, 1989
2. Bassett GAL, Mitchell SN, Gaston SA: Pulsing electromagnetic fields treatment in un-united fractures and failed arthrodesis. JAMA 247:623–628, 1982
3. Binder A, Hazelmann B, Parr P, et al: Pulsed electromagnetic field therapy on rotator cuff tendinitis. Lancet 1:695–698, 1984
4. Bonica JJ: The Management of Pain. Philadelphia, Lea & Febiger, 1990, pp 1850–1851
5. Carley P, Wainapel S: Electrotherapy for acceleration of wound healing: Low intensity direct current. Arch Phys Med Rehabil 66:443–446, 1985
6. Chantraine A, Ludy JP, Berger D: Is cortisone iontophoresis possible? Arch Phys Med Rehabil 67:38–40, 1986
7. DeLisa JA (ed): Rehabilitation Medicine: Principles and Practice. Philadelphia, JB Lippincott, 1988, pp 257–275
8. Deyo RA, Walsh NE, Martin DG, et al: A controlled trial of transcutaneous electrical nerve stimulation (TENS) and exercise for chronic low back pain. N Engl J Med 322:1627–1634, 1990
9. Duncombe A, Hopp JF: Modalities of physical treatment. Physical Medicine and Rehabilitation: State of the Art Reviews 5:493–519, 1991
10. Finney JW, et al: Low frequency transcutaneous nerve stimulation in reflex sympathetic dystrophy. Journal of Neurological and Orthopaedic Medicine and Surgery 12:270–273, 1991
11. Godfrey CM: Antihabituation: A new modality for chronic pain relief. Presented at the International Congress of Rehabilitation Medicine, Toronto, Canada, November 1988
12. Goldin JH, Broadbent NRG, Nancarrow JD: The effects of diapulse on the healing of wounds. Br J Plast Surg 34:267–270, 1981
13. Gritzer G, Arluke A: The Making of Rehabilitation: A Political Economy of Medical Specialization, 1890–1980. Berkeley, University of California Press, pp 1–37
14. Kottke JF, Lehmann JF: Krusen's Handbook of Physical Medicine and Rehabilitation, ed 4. Philadelphia, WB Saunders, 1990

15. Krusen FH: Physical Medicine: The Employment of Physical Agents for Diagnosis and Therapy. Philadelphia, WB Saunders, 1941, pp 22–35
16. Law JD: Percutaneous spinal cord stimulation for the "failed back surgery syndrome." Pain Management Update 1(1):1–2, 1990
17. Lee MHM, Laio SJ: Acupuncture in physiatry. In Kottke JF, Lehman JF (eds): Krusen's Handbook of Physical Medicine and Rehabilitation, ed 4. Philadelphia, WB Saunders, 1990, pp 402–432
18. Nagelschmidt KF: Specific effects of high frequency currents and magnetotherapy. British Journal of Physical Medicine 3:201–207, 1940
19. Nathan PW, Wall PD: Treatment of posthepatic neuralgia by prolonged electrical stimulation. Br Med J 3:645–647, 1974
20. Nippel FJ: Interferential current therapy: An advanced method in the management of pain. Presented at the American Physical Therapy Association Annual Conference, Atlanta, June 1979
21. Nolan FD, Barry G, Coughlan RJ: Pulsed high frequency electromagnetic therapy for persistent neck pain. Orthopedics 13:445, 1990
22. North RB, Ewend M, Lawton M, et al: Failed back surgery syndrome: 5-year follow-up after spinal cord stimulator implantation. Neurosurgery 28:692–699, 1991
23. Panel on Review of Neurological Devices, US Food and Drug Administration: Report on the Findings on Transcutaneous Electrical Nerve Stimulation for Pain Relief, February 1976
24. Pape KE, Galil A, Boulton JE, et al: Therapeutic electrical stimulation in the rehabilitation of children with cerebral palsy. Pediatr Res 23:6556A, 1988
25. Picher RI: Current trends: Low-volt pulsed microamp stimulation. Clinical Management 9:10–14, 28–33, 1989
26. Pomeranz B: Transcutaneous nerve stimulation. In Adman G (ed): Encyclopedia of Neuroscience. Boston, Birkhaven, 1987
27. Roberts HJ: TENS in the management of pancreatic pain. South Med J 71:396–399, 1978
28. Saal JA, Saal JS: Late stage management of lumbar spine problems. Physical Medicine and Rehabilitation Clinics of North America 2:205–222, 1991
29. Shealy CN: Biofeedback training in the physician's office: Transfer of pain clinic advances to primary care. Wis Med J 77:541–543, 1978
30. Shealy CN: Clinical observation—vitamin B6 and other vitamin levels in chronic pain patients. Clinical Journal of Pain 2:203–204, 1986
31. Shealy CN: Effects of transcranial neurostimulation upon mood and serotonin production: A preliminary report. Dolore 1:13–16, 1979
32. Shealy CN: Electrical stimulation of peripheral nerve, skin, and spinal cord for control of pain: Six and a half years' experience. Excerpta Medica International Congress Series 293:78, 1973
33. Shealy CN: The current status of dorsal column stimulation for relief of pain. In Wulfsohn NL, Sances A (eds): The Nervous System and Electrical Currents, vol 2. New York, Plenum Press, 1971, p 113
34. Shealy CN, Cady RK, Veehoff D, et al: The neurochemistry of depression. American Journal of Pain Management 2:13–16, 1992
35. Shealy CN, Cady RK, Wilkie RG, et al: Depression: A diagnostic, neurochemical profile & therapy with cranial electrical stimulation (CES). Journal of Neurological & Orthopaedic Medicine & Surgery 10:319–321, 1989
36. Shealy CN, Mortimer JT: Dorsal column electroanalgesia. In Reynolds DV, Sjoberg AE (eds): Neurological Research. Springfield, IL, Charles C Thomas, 1971
37. Sjolund BH, Eriksson M, Loersen JD: Transcutaneous and implanted electrical stimulation of peripheral nerves. In Bonica JJ (ed): Proceedings of the Third World Congress on Pain. (Advances in Pain Research and Theory, vol 5.) New York, Raven Press, 1983, pp 1852–1856
38. Sohn N, Weinstein MA, Robbins RD: The levator syndrome and its treatment with high voltage electrogalvanic stimulation. Am J Surg 144:580–582, 1982
39. Soloman RA, Viernstein MG, Donlem ML: Reduction of postoperative pain and narcotic use by transcutaneous electrical nerve stimulation. Surgery 87:142–146, 1980

40. Tulgar M, et al: Comparative effectiveness of different stimulation modes in relieving pain. Part I. A pilot study. Pain 47:151–155, 1991
41. Tulgar M, et al: Comparative effectiveness of different stimulation modes in relieving pain. Part II. A double-blind controlled long-term clinical trial. Pain 47:157–162, 1991
42. Tully TF, Schlesenger RC, Powell W, et al: Transcutaneous electrical nerve stimulations (TENS) devices. Report of the Office of Inspector General, United States Department of Health and Human Services, July 1990
43. Wilson DH: Treatment of soft tissue injuries by pulsed electrical energy. British Journal of Physical Medicine 1:269–270, 1972
44. Wolfe SL, Gersh MR, Rao VR: Examination of electrode placement and stimulating parameters in treating chronic pain with conventional transcutaneous electrical nerve stimulation (TENS). Pain 11:37–47, 1981

Address reprint requests to

Charles C. Mauldin, Jr, MD, PhD
3800 S. National Avenue, Suite 460
Springfield, MO 65807

PAIN CLINICS
What Type and When to Refer?

Donald F. Stanton, DO

Pain can, and often does, outlive its usefulness as an alarm system warning of actual or impending tissue damage. Simply stated, this is pain that our patients don't need. It is pain that can trigger exorbitant expenditures of money with repeated and escalating diagnostic efforts and seemingly never-ending attempts at treatment, all of which are ultimately exercises in futility. It is pain that can create horrendous suffering, extending beyond the patient to encompass the entire family. It is pain that can create unnecessary and prolonged disability, adding to the exorbitant cost through compensation payments, replacement services, lost wages, and overuse of the health care system. It is pain that can lead to an unhealthy lifestyle, with improper nutritional habits and inactivity. It is pain that frustrates the medical profession, employers, insurance carriers, the legal profession, legislative bodies, and, most of all, patients and their families. This is chronic pain.

As physicians, our first duty to all patients is to determine the cause of their presenting problem and to "cure" it, if we can. When we are not successful in that pursuit, it is then our duty to help relieve their pain and attendant suffering. For us to be effective in this role, we must have a clear understanding of the difference between the pain and the suffering.[13] Pain can be evaluated only on the basis of physical findings and by observing pain behavior. Pain behavior can be, and in chronic pain usually is, affected by several factors in addition to nociception. These factors include emotion, personality, beliefs, environment, and others. It should be kept in mind that our patient's complaint may not be our patient's problem. Both these duties must be performed in the context of maintaining and restoring the highest quality of lifestyle possible for our patients and their families. This aspect is too frequently dismissed as a social responsibility not within the physician's domain. The primary- and secondary-care physicians are theoretically in the best position to ensure high-quality, cost-effective care as well as the highest quality of lifestyle for his or her patients.

From the Department of Physical Medicine and Rehabilitation, College of Osteopathic Medicine, Michigan State University, East Lansing, Michigan

PHYSICAL MEDICINE AND REHABILITATION CLINICS
OF NORTH AMERICA

VOLUME 4 • NUMBER 1 • FEBRUARY 1993

The high financial and human cost of chronic pain is related to delayed diagnosis, prolonged nonproductive diagnostic procedures, repeated failure in nonspecific treatment and control methods, unnecessary suffering, and extended disability. Successful treatment of these syndromes demands an approach much different and with a wider purview than the traditional medical "find it, fix it, cure it" model with which physicians are so expert and successful in the management of acute pain syndromes. Those conventional medical procedures indicated for acute pain syndromes, if used in the treatment of chronic pain, are often ineffective and may in fact be iatrogenic.[17] Patients with painful conditions in which the cause is readily identified and amenable to effective treatment ("cured") are usually able to return to their former lifestyle, including work, as a routine matter without the need for further intervention. In those instances in which the cause is not clear, the treatment seems to be ineffective, or there is a continuation of pain and disability, prompt referral to a special center is indicated. Headaches and musculoskeletal syndromes, of which low back pain is predominant, commonly defy accurate diagnosis. Most of these syndromes are self-limiting with or without supportive treatment,[9, 10] and there should be little or no disability associated. If pain and disability continue beyond a reasonable time, e.g., 6 to 12 weeks, referral to a specialty center should be made promptly. The appropriate treatment of those with chronic pain can be very expensive; however, inappropriate treatment, delay in diagnosis, and prolonged suffering and disability are far more expensive.

WHAT IS CHRONIC PAIN?

This unnecessary persistent pain that has been designated as being chronic has been defined many ways. It has been commonly accepted that for a pain to be designated as chronic, it must be present for at least 6 months and, by more recent standards, 3 months.[24] These designations delay and hamper clinical management, because most acute pain problems heal within 3 or 4 weeks, at most 6 weeks. Appropriate clinical management would be facilitated if the diagnosis of chronic pain is entertained as early as 1 month beyond the expected healing time.[5] Etiologic factors other than nociception may be involved in maintaining the pain, pain behaviors, and suffering and should be considered in the management of these patients. Pain can also persist purely because of known continued or recurrent nociception in conditions such as arthritis and cancer, and nonnociceptive etiologic factors may also contribute to pain behaviors in these patients.

In those cases in which the nociceptive source cannot be identified, central factors possibly prolong the pain experience. These factors may be a result of nerve pathway degeneration seen with the deafferentation syndrome as a result of peripheral nerve injury[15, 16]; plastic changes in the central nervous system as a result of prolonged nociception[7, 29]; a result of a learning process resulting from environmental circumstances[12]; or any combination of these factors. Attributing the cause as "being all in the mind" is fallacious and serves no useful purpose in patient management.[12]

The common denominator of all chronic pain patients is the constant or recurrent experience of unrelenting pain. There is a duality to pain, with two operational components: sensory-discriminative and affective-motivational.[23] The sensory-discriminative component deals with the process of localization and identification of the nociceptive source. The pain detection threshold is a part of this component. The motivational-affective component concerns the feelings that arise from the unpleasant sensation, which creates a desire to escape. Pain tolerance is part of this component. The pain detection threshold is fairly constant within an individual and among different individuals. Pain tolerance, on the other hand, is demonstrated by great variability in the suffering and anxiety among individuals with seemingly same stimuli and is dependent on personality traits and situational factors.[11] I have long suspected that more people experience chronic pain than physicians realize. Some believe that the pain that they experience is expected by virtue of their activities or age and do not believe that medicine has anything to offer. Others may come to this conclusion after one or more unsuccessful efforts to obtain relief. Some may be in a position to adjust their activities and lifestyles to accommodate their chronic pain and thus improve their tolerance. I refer to this group as the "silent sufferers." There may be a greater motive to reporting pain than simply seeking relief. The complaint could well be an attempt on the part of the patient to improve the situation in which he or she finds him or herself. The Boeing study reported that low-level job satisfaction may be the most important determinant in reporting lower back pain,[3] which suggests that some people who do not report low back pain may have a higher degree of job satisfaction, which increases their tolerance. If this situation is not recognized, the worker and the health care system may be victimized, leading to increased suffering of the worker, needless liability on the part of the physician or surgeon, and unnecessary expenditure of health care dollars.

Chronic pain is most often described as a deep aching, burning-type pain, in contrast to the sharp, pricking quality of acute pain. The patient's affect does not appear to be consistent with the high level of pain intensity reported on the pain scales. Exacerbations occur with varying frequency and intensity. The activity level fluctuates widely; the patient may be fully active or bedridden. Chronic pain can produce a symptom complex characterized by a series of behaviors denoting that misinformation, misperceptions, and environmental situations have resulted in a suffering state and, frequently, unwarranted disability. These behaviors include

multiple verbal and nonverbal complaints of pain (bodily preoccupation)
absence from the work place
restricted physical activity (invalidism)
inconsistent physical performance
improper dietary habits
inappropriate drug usage (analgesic abuse)
doctor shopping
searching for alternative methods of treatment and quackery
increased alcohol consumption
depression or anxiety
multiple organ complaints without objective diagnoses, e.g., functional cardiac and gastrointestinal disorders
temporary relief of as long as 3 months with each new treatment attempt (placebo or endorphin effect)
requesting surgery, the "quick fix"
overuse or manipulation of the medical care system.

These behaviors lead to a conviction of illness, physical deconditioning, loss of self-esteem, weight gain, low energy level, lack of motivation, marital discord, unemployability, financial difficulties, hopelessness, frustration, and loss of self-control.

These behaviors are commonly and mistakenly attributed to malingering or to attempts to obtain secondary gain. Many of these are learned behaviors and are under environmental influence.[12] These behaviors begin with the initial incident and are reinforced by the ensuing medical care and subsequent bureaucratic and legal morass. There is a cognitive component affecting this behavior resulting from a lack of understanding of the medical condition, employer, insurance, and legal issues. This lack of understanding may be due to inadequate, incorrect, or conflicting explanations. It may also be due to the patient's impaired ability to process correct and complete information. This impaired ability may be because of lowered intellect[21] or cognitive deficits such as impaired memory or concentration and poor judgment as a result of a learning disability or traumatic brain injury.[1, 19] These same cognitive deficits may, however, be seen as a result of the chronic pain itself. Differentiation is often difficult and may require neuropsychological evaluation. The problems are many and complex. In varying degree, they encompass medical, psychological, social, financial, vocational, and avocational issues.

WHY REFER TO A PAIN CLINIC?

Many patients with chronic pain do not have a discernible cause of nociception[22] but deserve appropriate medical management. First, the diagnostic effort should be appropriate and completed without delay, probably over a period no longer than 3 months. Nonspecific treatment or pain-control methods should be restricted to noninvasive modalities and monitored closely for effectiveness. It should always be kept in mind that the placebo effect of any new treatment with the hope of cure or relief can be successful in the short term.[8] The pain then often returns with a vengeance, frequently with more profound depression and hopelessness. In our experience, any of these modalities is doomed to failure unless there is concurrent physical reconditioning and restoration of the former lifestyle, including return to work. When persistent or recurrent pain begins to have a life of its own and unwarranted suffering and disability appear, medical management must be redirected. Efforts must now shift from the diagnostic, treatment, and curative theme to the control of pain, suffering, and disability.

The distinction between pain and suffering becomes particularly important in back pain. It is with back pain that the confounding of pain with suffering, and suffering with disability, becomes the greatest. This confounding is true of the health care system, of agency and legal systems, and of the public. The result is often unnecessary disability.[13]

The clinician should assume that this milestone has been reached when pain persists 1 month beyond the time expected for healing to occur or when pain reoccurs without cause.[5]

The treating physician must be confident and comfortable with the diagnosis of chronic pain with an unknown cause. It is incumbent on the physician to explain this entity accurately to the patient, spouse, family, and significant others in terms that they can readily understand. This area is often where the art of medicine is critical. Some patients can learn with a simple explanation, but others must learn by trial and error. In gaining this understanding, it may be necessary for the physician to spend an inordinate amount of time with much repetition and support. Hurt must be distinguished from harm, and pain must be distinguished from suffering.[12, 13] The reporting of pain without the occurrence of actual or impending tissue damage has a distinctly different connotation than the reporting of pain that is commensurate and consistent with tissue damage. The former is a symptom of the motivational-affective component of the pain experience, and the latter is a symptom of the sensory-discriminative component. This distinction drives the direction of medical care, with tissue damage primarily requiring specific treatment and pain-control modalities, whereas without ongoing tissue damage, suffering, psychological reaction, and environmental factors must be addressed. Early return to activity, especially at the work site, is important to prevent psychosocial deterioration and unnecessary disability. Behavioral psychological counseling may be necessary, as may vocational rehabilitation services. Appropriate providers of these services should be identified within the community and monitored by the physician for their effectiveness in the restoration of an independent lifestyle. All should understand that even if the pain cannot be cured or relieved, the suffering and disability can be. Some patients develop a suffering state with chronic pain behavior in response to their beliefs and personal circumstances, resulting in a prolonged disability. These individuals consume enormous financial resources and adversely affect their own health and the well-being of their immediate family. If this symptom complex becomes ingrained, a comprehensive rehabilitation effort is most likely necessary.

SETTING RESTRICTIONS

Physicians are frequently called on to delineate specific activities that their patient is unable to perform. Simple forms are usually provided, and it is expected that they be completed. These forms address only physical ability. In some cases, this procedure is appropriate if there is a well-defined physical problem, e.g., amputation; there has been prolonged absence from the workplace; and the same job, with the same employer and co-workers, is available with only minimal accommodation. In many conditions, and especially with chronic pain syndromes, the ability to perform physically is compromised by the patient's belief system[2, 21, 25, 27]: "Can't I really be cured?" "Can't this pain be relieved?" "Will this activity cause me more harm?" "Will I become crippled?" "Will this job cause me more pain?" "Will I be treated fairly?" "Will I be laid off or fired?" "Can I sustain the activity 8 hours a day, 5 days a week?" and so on. These are real concerns, and because others (doctors, employers, insurance companies) believe that they are not a problem, the patient may believe that they are and very often does so. Self-esteem, self-confidence, job satisfaction, and a social environment at the work site are additional factors. Performance is also affected according to the individual's mood or emotional state at any given time and thus has a profound effect on pain tolerance. Chronic-pain patients are most consistent in their inconsistency. We have an axiom that "some days they can lick a bull and some days they can't lick a postage stamp." These issues and others must be assessed and considered in determining restrictions if the goal is truly to be successful in assisting them in returning to a meaningful, gainful employment sustained over time.

Typically, restrictions are developed by the physician, estimating what the patient cannot do. Some may actually ask the patient what he or she cannot do. There is also machine testing, often with a computer, which makes beautiful graphs and reports that "objectively" determine physical ability. Some try to predict what activities exacerbate the chronic pain, and some try to actually predict what activities cause further tissue damage. The final decision is, however, arrived at by what the physician believes. If there is a wide disparity between what the physician believes and what the patient believes, the return-to-work effort will most surely fail. Obviously, if this does occur, it usually is the patient's fault and sole responsibility. This system solves everybody's problem except the worker's and his or her family's. They are often branded as malingerers, secondary gainers, unmotivated, uncooperative, less-than-solid citizens, low-back "losers," and so on.

Restrictions, if they are to have any semblance of reality with chronic pain patients, must consider all of the following three points:

physical capability
prevention of tissue damage
activity tolerance.

Physical capability should consider age, sex, strength, range of motion, endurance, repetitiveness, position, and balance. These factors can be assessed several ways, but we must always be mindful of our limitations and objectivity. In other words, we may be wrong. Prevention of tissue damage is a purely medical decision, and the correct one often may not be truly known except over time. The physician must distinguish between what only hurts and what does actual harm. Again, we may be wrong. Activity tolerance secondary to chronic pain is purely subjective and must be determined solely by the patient. There are cases in which the patient appears to have the physical capability to perform a particular job and there is no objective evidence of tissue damage, yet the patient is unable to tolerate the required level of activity to sustain an adequate job performance. This incongruity must be explored more deeply by the physician and treating team, as must a true understanding of our patient's beliefs and the social work environment in which the worker is to be placed. The social work environment includes the attitudes and beliefs of the co-workers, supervisors, employer, and so on. Again, we and the patient may be wrong. The bottom line, then, is that the physician must direct a comprehensive assessment, and the treatment and rehabilitation effort must extend beyond medical, surgical, and physical therapy care.[28] The patient's beliefs must be assessed and an effort made to correct beliefs that are inappropriate and preventing full function. The physician must also assess his or her own beliefs and correct those that are inappropriate. There are times in which the social environment at the job site prevents return to work or staying at the job. I often ascribe a worker's inability to perform a specific job as due to his or her perception of pain. These social factors are more important than the physical requirements (in the absence of tissue damage—hurt versus harm) in successful and permanent placement. I usually recommend return to work with minimal on no restriction, because setting restrictions gives the patient the message that activity does harm. I cannot predict what activity produces the perception of pain.

I am biased that we as physicians should refuse to delineate restrictions and should delineate only the ability to perform a series of tasks or a specific job. I am convinced that trial and error in a cooperative and informed atmosphere of all interested parties is the best policy. If we are able to solve our patient's problem, we have solved everybody's problem.

If the physician as authority figure tells a patient that he or she is unable to do something, the patient will not do it because of the expectation of pain,[2] especially at work, even though the patient may know full well it can be done. This creates confusion and distrust toward the physician on the part of the patient. In my experience, restrictions are used more often to keep my patients from getting a job than to help them to do so.

Until the medical profession ceases to pontificate and to engrave our learned pronouncements in stone, many injured workers with chronic pain will continue to be outcasts of society. Needless suffering and economic ruin to the workers, their families, and society will continue unabated.

WHAT KIND OF PAIN CLINICS ARE AVAILABLE?

Five issues require consideration in the management of painful syndromes:

diagnosis
definitive treatment
control of pain
suffering
disability.

There are several types of pain-treatment facilities, each accepting diagnostic categories and using treatment techniques that are usually dependent on the practitioner involved. Pain-treatment programs are designed to deal with one or more of these issues. Although all of the issues are considered in every pain program to some extent, there is usually a predominant focus on one or two.

The following is a guide to help the physician assess the type of facility with which he or she is dealing. The categories used are this author's and are based on outcome or goal orientation. Most facilities do not label themselves accordingly.

Diagnosis-and-Treatment-of-Pain Clinics

Patients with pain that persists despite the best diagnostic and treatment effort of the local medical facilities and might benefit from further investigation deserve referral to a specialized pain diagnosis-and-treatment center. These major centers should have an organized multidisciplinary staff that functions in close cooperation, focusing on each patient's situation. These centers should have a strong teaching-and-research component and are usually affiliated with a university. There are excellent pain clinics, which may or may not be part of a major center, that specialize in specific diagnoses such as headache, low back pain, and arthritis. These clinics require only two or three disciplines to be effective. Caution is to be exercised when pain-treatment clinics that use single modalities, e.g., biofeedback, acupuncture, and trigger point injections, are considered. If the only tool available is a hammer, everything looks like a nail.

Pain-Control Clinics

Clinics that specialize in the control of pain are usually staffed by anesthesiologists. The mainstay of treatment consists of nerve blocks, transcutaneous nerve stimulation units, medications, epidural injections, intrathecal infusions, and other innovative methods of analgesia. Surgical procedures may be offered in the form of peripheral nerve, spinal cord, and brain stimulators. Effectiveness depends on the success of interruption of the transmission of pain impulses from objectively identified sources of nociception, e.g., cancer or areas of delayed healing.

Diagnosis-and-treatment pain clinics and pain-control pain facilities primarily target the sensory-discriminative aspects of the pain experience. Expected outcomes are identification of the origin and effective treatment that "cures" and thus relieves the pain; identification of the origin, determining that effective treatment and "cure" are not possible and providing a basis for prescribing effective pain-control measures; and making the determination that the cause cannot be identified or that effective control is not possible.

If successful pain control is achieved, the side effects of the method must be evaluated in the context of a high-quality, meaningful lifestyle. The patient may opt for less pain control in a tradeoff for being able to participate in the enjoyment of life. For example, some modalities are cerebral depressants that may be unpleasant for the patient, or the mode of delivery, such as intrathecal infusions, may not allow comfortable, dignified community participation. Another issue may be unwillingness or fear of undergoing a procedure such as the implantation of a spinal cord or brain stimulator. These wishes should be respected without passing of judgment and labeling of the patient as uncooperative, unmotivated, or malingering.

Psychological Pain Clinics

Psychological pain programs are usually staffed by psychologists or psychiatrists. Various techniques and modalities are used to address coping, relaxation, and stress management. Biofeedback, hypnosis, and imaging techniques may be useful. Behavioral modification approaches are frequently incorporated. The patient's belief systems and the external forces in the environment causing misconceptions and chronic pain behaviors that lead to disproportionate disability are addressed. These clinics target the motivational-affective aspect of the pain experience, with the expectation that relief of suffering is sufficient to restore the patient to a physically active, rewarding lifestyle. Inappropriate physical restrictions placed by physicians who lack an understanding of disability may hamper successful outcome in these types of clinics.

Work-Hardening Pain Clinics

Work-hardening facilities emphasize physical conditioning, although some psychological support is usually provided. Tasks are developed with repetitive activities over a 6 to 8-hour period, with the goal of developing strength and endurance. This approach seems to be effective and appropriate for those individuals recovering from an acute problem who have not had prolonged disability[26] and whose previous job was satisfying and available. There is the possibility that the work-hardening environment is such that return to work becomes an attractive escape. It has been our experience that the social environment at the work site is at least as important, if not more so, than the physical requirements of the job in determining successful return to work. Individual physical examination and biomechanical measures do not predict future employment status when controlled for age and length of disability.[14] As a general rule, chronic-pain patients with well-developed pain behaviors and prolonged disability do not respond well to this type of approach.

Disability or Functional Restoration Pain Clinics

Programs that address the multiple aspects of pain use multidisciplinary or interdisciplinary team treatment, including psychology, physical therapy, and vocational counseling. These clinics must be eclectic in their approach. Diagnostic, treatment, and control efforts should be minimal. Suffering is addressed in much the same way as in psychological clinics, with techniques that allow the patient to be an active participant socially and vocationally. Physical restrictions and abilities are determined by a physician knowledgeable in the area of disability. Patients appropriate for this type of clinic include those with persistent pain in whom it has been determined that physical activity is not contraindicated.

Expected outcomes include

physically active, high-quality lifestyle
gainful employment as indicated
restrictions based on harm, not hurt
a proper medication regimen
appropriate usage of the health care system.

General Considerations

A pain-treatment facility that has the appropriate disciplines, expertise, adequate facilities and equipment, and the concept necessary not only to relieve the pain when possible but to restore the patient to a high-quality, independent lifestyle with return to full activity, including work, must be identified. Obtaining pain relief facilitates the process but is not a prerequisite to a successful outcome. This concept is the realization that the pain reported by the patient has cognitive, affective, and environmental origins in addition to those caused by body damage. The pain clinic must also treat the associated disability in addition to the pain experience.[21]

It is difficult for any program to be all things to all people. The patient may require more than one type of program for a recovery process to be ultimately successful. When the pain facility is to be chosen, the appropriate type should be determined by an assessment of the patient's needs. Failure of one type of pain facility does not preclude success in another. Some clinics seem to treat their patients according to the staff's expertise and skill, and others seem to be driven by the ability to be adequately reimbursed. Many times, this is without fully considering the effects on the patient, which at times can be devastating.

The practitioner should evaluate the programs available and should not necessarily expect a certain outcome because of the facility's name. Calling a horse a zebra does not give it stripes. The International Association for the Study of Pain, through a task force, has published a monograph defining the desirable characteristics for pain treatment facilities. (See end of article.)

Chronic pain may be treated in inpatient or outpatient facilities. Inpatient programs have the advantage of high-level technology and subspecialty multidisciplinary expertise congregated at one location. Total environmental control is possible, which may be necessary to treat drug withdrawal, alcoholism, and severe pain behaviors, such as inability to ambulate, effectively. Inpatient programs are expensive; additionally, there may be difficulty in transferring the newly learned behavior from the hospital to the home, community, and vocational environments.[27]

Outpatient programs often address the same issues as in inpatient programs; however, the patient is in his or her usual environment. Community reintegration may be more effective, and there may be a lower incidence of relapse. These programs may be more cost effective in that expensive lodging need not be provided. Behavioral change may be more difficult and take longer because of lack of environmental control. Programs that continue from an inpatient component to an outpatient component have an obvious benefit in selected cases and may at times be the most appropriate.

TEAM TREATMENT

Individuals with a myriad of problems create a complexity in treatment and rehabilitation that exceeds the ability of any individual practitioner to provide. Team care for patients with pain problems was pioneered by Bonica.[6] There has been a recognition that the medical model is inadequate and inefficient in providing the necessary services required when multiple providers are involved.[6, 18] There are distinctions between multidisciplinary teams and interdisciplinary teams that should be understood.[18]

The multidisciplinary team is based on the medical consultation model. The physician determines the need for each particular discipline and consults with each individually. Each team member focuses on goals that pertain to his or her particular discipline. Information is provided in a vertical direction to the prescribing physician, who then makes decisions about the global goals of the patient and assesses progress and the need for further intervention. This communication is provided individually by report or through team conferences on a formal or informal basis. This team can be managed by a physician in practice and is effective for patients recovering from an acute problem that has not been complicated by psychosocial issues.

The interdisciplinary team, in contrast, is assembled by the physician, but each discipline participates in planning the services to be provided and in establishing the global goals for the patient. The goals within each discipline are then developed and complement each of the other disciplines, leading toward the overall patient goal. Communication is horizontal, with each team member equal to the physician, who is also an integral member of the team. This approach is difficult, if not impossible, to manage in outpatients with a solo practitioner.

In the rehabilitation setting, with a stable patient, medical care of a diagnostic or treatment nature plays a lesser role; however, monitoring of the medical condition is vital to the success of team management. "In the eyes of the patient, the physician legitimates the entire program."[21]

The team should be composed of the necessary disciplines, including a physician knowledgeable in rehabilitation, such as a physiatrist; other medical or surgical specialists; nurses; a physical therapist; an occupational therapist; a psychologist; a neuropsychologist; a nutritionist; an exercise physiologist; a speech and language pathologist; a social worker; a vocational rehabilitation counselor; and others deemed appropriate.

It is helpful for the referring physician to have a thorough understanding of the patient's problem and needs and to have formulated an expected outcome goal. A pain facility that encompasses the expertise, the resources, and the proper concepts to achieve the expected outcome goal must then be identified. The referring physician should expect to be kept informed of the progress of his or her patient, should have a general understanding of the process, and should cooperate with and augment the treatment and rehabilitation plan to maintain consistency throughout the patient's environment. Questions and concerns should be freely discussed with the program director or the attending physician. Expressing these questions and concerns to the patient and family may cause doubt and may interfere with the overall progress or even ensure failure. It must be recognized that some of the approaches used in pain clinics are nontraditional and may not seem consistent with the excellent training received in the medical model. Failure to adhere to these principles most often creates confusion and distrust with the program and dooms the outcome to failure.

Patients afflicted with persistent pain deserve appropriate, effective treatment. They should not be dismissed as malingerers, secondary gainers, crooks, kooks, or as people who are not solid citizens. By the same token, medical care providers should accept that it is often difficult and sometimes impossible to diagnose, treat, and rehabilitate these people adequately. To improve our effectiveness, the team approach using several disciplines is necessary. Probably even more important is the need to provide education to change the attitudes of employers, insurers, the legal system, and physicians as it pertains to the care of individuals in whom objective evidence does not substantiate their complaints.

SPECIFICS IN THE TREATMENT OF CHRONIC PAIN OF UNKNOWN ORIGIN

Chronic-pain patients who present with pain behaviors and inappropriate levels of disability require management by a physician who interacts with the patient as if the following tenets were true:

The pain is real
The pain is not curable
Only about 1% eventually have a documented origin for their pain
Pain perception can change
There is an effective endogenous pain-inhibitory system
Medications and modalities such as transcutaneous nerve stimulation units may be more of a hindrance than a help
Physical activity may, and probably will, hurt but will not harm
Pain perception lessens with meaningful, enjoyable activity
Patients need to be needed.

Always keep in mind Fordyce's law: "People who have something better to do, don't suffer as much."[13]

References

1. Anderson JM, Kaplan MS, Felsenthal G: Brain injury obscured by chronic pain: A preliminary report. Arch Phys Med Rehabil 71:703–708, 1990
2. Bayer TL, Baer PE, Early C: Situational and psychophysiological factors in psychologically induced pain. Pain 44:45–50, 1991
3. Bigos SJ, Battie MC, Spengler DM, et al: A prospective study of work perceptions and psychosocial factors affecting the report of back injury. Spine 16:1–6, 1991
4. Bigos SJ, Andary MT: Practitioner's guide to industrial back problems. Neurosurgery Clinics of North America 2:863–875, 1991
5. Bonica JJ: General considerations of chronic pain. In Bonica JJ (ed): The Management of Pain, vol 1, ed 2. Philadelphia, Lea & Febiger, 1990, p 180
6. Bonica JJ: Evolution and current status of pain programs. Journal of Pain and Symptom Management 5:368–374, 1990
7. Britton NF, Skevington SM: A mathematical model of the gate control theory of pain. J Theor Biol 137:91–105, 1989
8. Chapman SL, Brena SF: Pain and society. Annals of Behavioral Medicine 7:21–24, 1985
9. Dillane JB, Fry J, Kalton G: Acute back syndrome—a study from general practice. Br Med J 3:82–84, 1966
10. Dixon AS: Introduction. In Jayson MIV (ed): The Lumbar Spine and Back Pain. Tunbridge Wells, Pitman Medical, 1980, pp 1–28
11. Fields HL: Pain. New York, McGraw-Hill, 1987
12. Fordyce WE: Psychological factors in the failed back. Int Disabil Stud 10:29–31, 1988
13. Fordyce WE: Pain and suffering: A reappraisal. Am Psychol 43:276–283, 1988

14. Gallagher RM, Rauh V, Haugh LD, et al: Determinants of return-to-work among low back pain patients. Pain 39:55–67, 1989

15. Gobel S: An electron microscopic analysis of trans-synaptic effects of peripheral nerve injury subsequent to tooth pulp extirpations on neurons in laminae I and II of the medullary dorsal horn. Journal of Neurosci 4:2281–2290, 1984

16. Gobel S, Binck JM: Degenerative changes in primary trigeminal exons and in neurons in nucleus caudillos following tooth pulp extirpations in the cat. Brain Res 132:347–354, 1977

17. Gottlieb HJ, Alperson BL, Koller R, et al: An innovative program for the restoration of patients with chronic back pain. Journal of the American Physical Therapy Association 59:996–999, 1979

18. Howard ME: Interdisciplinary team treatment in acute care. *In* Deutsch PM, Fralish KM: Innovations in Head Injury Rehabilitation. New York, Matthew Bender, 1988, pp 160–186

19. Janda V: Muscles, central nervous motor regulation and back problems. *In* Korr I (ed): Neurobiologic Mechanisms in Manipulative Therapy. New York, Plenum, 1978

20. Jensen MP, Turner JA, Romano JM: Self-efficacy and outcome expectancies: Relationship to chronic pain coping strategies and adjustment. Pain 44:263–269, 1991

21. Loeser JD: The role of pain clinics in managing chronic back pain. *In* Frymoyer JW (ed): The Adult Spine: Principles and Practice. New York, Raven Press, 1991

22. Loeser JD: What is chronic pain. Theor Med 12:213–225, 1991

23. Melzack R, Casey KL: Sensory, motivational, and central control determinants of pain: A new conceptual model. *In* Kenshalo D (ed): The Skin Senses. Springfield, IL, Charles C Thomas, 1968, pp 423–439

24. Merskey H: Classification of chronic pain. Pain Supplement 3, 1986

25. Slater MA, Hall HF, Atkinson JH, et al: Pain and impairment beliefs in chronic low back pain: Validation of the Pain and Impairment Relationship Scale (PAIRS). Pain 44:51–56, 1991

26. Tollison CD, Kriegel ML, Satterthwaite JR, et al: Comprehensive pain center treatment of low back worker's compensation injuries: An industrial medicine clinical outcome follow-up comparison. Orthop Rev 18:1115–1126, 1989

27. Turk DC, Rudy TE: Neglected topics in the treatment of chronic pain patients—relapse, noncompliance, and adherence enhancement. Pain 44:5–28, 1991

28. Waddell G, Pilowsky I, Bond MR: Clinical assessment and interpretation of abnormal illness behavior in low back pain. Pain 39:41–53, 1989

29. Willis WW Jr: The Pain System. Basel, S. Karger, 1985

Address reprint requests to

Donald F. Stanton, DO
Department of Physical Medicine and Rehabilitation
College of Osteopathic Medicine
Michigan State University
B401 West Fee Hall
East Lansing, MI 48824

Desirable Characteristics for Pain Treatment Facilities

Facilities for the treatment of patients with chronic pain have developed rapidly in the past fifteen years. There have been few, if any, governmental or professional standards or controls for such patient care facilities, even in the developed nations of the world. In the United States of America, pain treatment facilities that exist within hospitals are theoretically evaluated under the aegis of the Joint Committee on the Accreditation of Hospitals, but the accreditation process does not specifically assess the pain treatment facility. Free-standing pain treatment programs and those within hospitals may also obtain voluntary certification from the Commission on Accreditation of Rehabilitation Facilities through a program instituted with assistance from the American Pain Society in 1983. In other countries, both governmental agencies and the national chapters of the International Association for the Study of Pain (IASP) have developed some standards. Governmental health care systems in some countries regulate all aspects of the provision of health care, and the freedom to establish new types of health care delivery is limited.

The International Association for the Study of Pain believes that patients throughout the world would benefit from the establishment of a set of desirable characteristics for pain treatment facilities. Although IASP itself does not plan to offer certification or accreditation, the standards set forth in this document can serve as a guideline for both practitioners and those governmental or professional organizations involved in the establishment of standards for this type of health care delivery. The field of pain management has been viewed with skepticism by many physicians and health policy and funding administrators; reasonable guidelines should be established and adhered to by reputable treatment facilities.

It is important to recognize that not every patient referred to a pain treatment facility requires the services of a large number of health care professionals. Nonetheless, many pain patients do require the services of multiple disciplines and resources must be available to effectively manage the patient. It is on the basis of the types of resources available that the following classification scheme has been proposed.

This Task Force has not addressed the issues of pain management in the post-operative or post-trauma setting. Such treatment programs may occur within a pain treatment facility, but they are not required for the assessment and treatment of patients with chronic pain.

This document has been prepared by a Task Force appointed by the President of IASP, Dr. Michael J. Cousins, and chaired by the Secretary of IASP, Dr. John D. Loeser.

From Loeser JD: Desirable Characteristics for Pain Treatment Facilities. Seattle, International Association for the Study of Pain, 1990; reprinted with permission of the International Association for the Study of Pain.

Definition of Terms

The following terms will be briefly defined in this section; a more complete description of the characteristics of each type of facility appears in subsequent portions of this report.

1. Pain treatment facility: A generic term used to describe all forms of pain treatment facilities without regard to personnel involved or types of patients served. Pain unit is a synonym for pain treatment facility.
2. Multidisciplinary pain center: An organization of health care professionals and basic scientists which includes research, teaching and patient care related to acute and chronic pain. This is the largest and most complex of the pain treatment facilities and ideally would exist as a component of a medical school or teaching hospital. Clinical programs must be supervised by an appropriately trained and licensed clinical director; a wide array of health care specialists is required, such as physicians, psychologists, nurses, physical therapists, occupational therapists, vocational counselors, social workers and other specialized health care providers.

   The disciplines of health care providers required is a function of the varieties of patients seen and the health care resources of the community. The members of the treatment team must communicate with each other on a regular basis, both about specific patients and about overall development. Health care services in a multidisciplinary pain clinic must be integrated and based upon multidisciplinary assessment and management of the patient. Inpatient and outpatient programs are offered in such a facility.
3. Multidisciplinary pain clinic: A health care delivery facility staffed by physicians of different specialties and other non-physician health care providers who specialize in the diagnosis and management of patients with chronic pain. This type of facility differs from a Multidisciplinary Pain Center only because it does not include research and teaching activities in its regular programs. A Multidisciplinary pain clinic may have diagnostic and treatment facilities which are outpatient, inpatient or both.
4. Pain clinic: A health care delivery facility focusing upon the diagnosis and management of patients with chronic pain. A pain clinic may specialize in specific diagnoses or in pains related to a specific region of the body. A pain clinic may be large or small but it should never be a label for an isolated solo practitioner. A single physician functioning within a complex health care institution which offers appropriate consultative and therapeutic services could qualify as a pain clinic, if chronic pain patients were suitably assessed and managed. The absence of interdisciplinary assessment and management distinguishes this type of facility from a multidisciplinary pain center or clinic. Pain clinics can, and should be encouraged to, carry out research, but it is not a required characteristic of this type of facility.
5. Modality-oriented clinic: This is a health care facility which offers a specific type of treatment and does not provide comprehensive assessment or management. Examples include nerve block clinic, transcutaneous nerve stimulation clinic, acupuncture clinic, biofeedback clinic, etc. Such a facility may have one or more health care providers with

different professional training; because of its limited treatment options and the lack of an integrated, comprehensive approach, it does not qualify for the term, multidisciplinary.

Desirable Characteristics of Multidisciplinary Pain Centers

1. A multidisciplinary pain center (MPC) should have on its staff a variety of health care providers capable of assessing and treating physical, psychosocial, medical, vocational and social aspects of chronic pain. These can include physicians, nurses, psychologists, physical therapists, occupational therapists, vocational counselors, social workers and any other type of health care professional who can make a contribution to patient diagnosis or treatment.

2. At least three medical specialties should be represented on the staff of a multidisciplinary pain center. If one of the physicians is not a psychiatrist, physicians from two specialities and a clinical psychologist are the minimum required. A multidisciplinary pain center must be able to assess and treat both the physical and the psychosocial aspects of a patient's complaints. The need for other types of health care providers should be determined on the basis of the population served by the MPC.

3. The health care professionals should communicate with each other on a regular basis both about individual patients and the programs which are offered in the pain treatment facility.

4. There should be a Director or Coordinator of the MPC. He or she needs not be a physician, but if not, there should be a Director of Medical Services who will be responsible for monitoring of the medical services provided.

5. The MPC should offer diagnostic and therapeutic services which include medication management, referral for appropriate medical consultation, review of prior medical records and diagnostic tests, physical examination, psychological assessment and treatment, physical therapy vocational assessment and counseling and other facilities as appropriate.

6. The MPC should have a designated space for its activities. The MPC should include facilities for inpatient services and outpatient services.

7. The MPC should maintain records on its patients so as to be able to assess individual treatment outcomes and to evaluate overall program effectiveness.

8. The MPC should have adequate support staff to carry out its activities.

9. Health care providers active in an MPC should have appropriate knowledge of both the basic sciences and clinical practices relevant to chronic pain patients.

10. The MPC should have a medically trained professional available to deal with patient referrals and emergencies.

11. All health care providers in an MPC should be appropriately licensed in the country or state in which they practice.

12. The MPC should be able to deal with a wide variety of chronic pain patients, including those with pain due to cancer and pain due to other diseases.

13. An MPC should establish protocols for patient management and assess their efficacy periodically.

14. An MPC should see an adequate number and variety of patients for its professional staff to maintain their skills in diagnosis and treatment.
15. Members of an MPC should be carrying out research on chronic pain. This does not mean that everyone should be doing both research and patient care. Some will only function in one arena, but the institution should have ongoing research activities.
16. The MPC should be active in educational programs for a wide variety of health care providers, including undergraduate, graduate and post-doctoral levels.
17. The MPC should be part of or closely affiliated with a major health sciences educational or research institution.

Desirable Characteristics for a Multidisciplinary Pain Clinic

The distinction between a Multidisciplinary Pain Center and a Multidisciplinary Pain Clinic is that the former has research and teaching components that need not be present in the latter. Hence, items #15, 16 and 17 above are not required for a Multidisciplinary Pain Clinic. All of the other items should be present.

Desirable Characteristics for a Pain Clinic

1. A Pain Clinic should have access to and regular interaction with at least three types of medical specialties or health care providers. If one of the physicians is not a psychiatrist, a clinical psychologist is essential.
2. The health care providers should communicate with each other on a regular basis both about individual patients and programs offered in the pain treatment facility.
3. There should be a Director or Coordinator of the Pain Clinic. If he or she is not a physician, there should be a Director of Medical Services who is responsible for the monitoring of medical services which are provided to the patients.
4. The Pain Clinic should offer both diagnostic and therapeutic services.
5. The Pain Clinic should have designated space for its activities.
6. The Pain Clinic should maintain records on its patients so as to be able to assess individual treatment outcomes and to evaluate overall program effectiveness.
7. The Pain Clinic should have adequate support staff to carry out its activities.
8. Health care providers working in a Pain Clinic should have appropriate knowledge of both the basic sciences and clinical practices relevant to pain patients.
9. The Pain Clinic should have a trained health care professional available to deal with patient referrals and emergencies.
10. All health care providers in a Pain Clinic should be appropriately licensed in the country and state in which they practice.

Discussion

The Task Force is strongly committed to the idea that a multidisciplinary approach to diagnosis and treatment is the preferred method of delivering health care to patients with chronic pain of any etiology. Not every patient referred to a pain treatment facility is in need of multidisciplinary diagnosis or treatment, but the facility should have those resources available when they are appropriate. Although the Task Force recognizes that health care resources are not uniformly distributed throughout any country or the world and that compromises will be necessary, all health care providers should strive to attain the standards set forth in this document for the care of patients with chronic pain. Health care providers in pain treatment facilities should be encouraged and expected to be members of IASP and its national chapters in order to facilitate exchange of information and research facilities.

The primary goal for a pain treatment facility is to provide effective, humane care for those who suffer from chronic pain. The complexities of the chronic pain patient must be recognized to accomplish these goals. In the modern era, however, the issue of cost effectiveness must also be considered and we cannot erect standards for chronic pain treatment which are above and beyond the standards for patients with other types of complaints. Moreover, health care delivery systems are rapidly changing and standards that prevent innovation and progress should not be proposed.

All patients with chronic pain should be appropriately evaluated before treatment is implemented. Facilities that offer only one type of treatment or have limited access to professionals in various disciplines must demonstrate appropriate patient selection prior to the initiation of therapy. Patients who attend such a health care facility should have been fully evaluated elsewhere before such a referral is made. For example, if a "pain clinic" specializes in headache patients and offers only biofeedback therapy, the patients referred to such a facility must have an appropriate medical evaluation prior to embarking on this treatment program. Pain treatment facilities must go beyond this stereotypic approach and determine what services the patient needs prior to embarking upon one or another type of treatment. If what the patient needs is not available, the patient should be referred elsewhere.

Resources and patient demands vary throughout the world, and there is no single guideline that can be made which well apply to every location. In developing nations, pain treatment facilities may appropriately consist of a small number of health care professionals with limited resources. Such groups may mainly see chronic pain due to cancer or to nervous system injuries; the problems of chronic pain as seen in the industrialized nations may have not yet arrived. Treatments may be limited to nerve blocks and drugs if economic conditions preclude more expensive treatment strategies. It is unlikely that research activities will be carried out in such an environment, but the mission of teaching other health care providers should never be overlooked.

In the developed nations of the world, there would seem to be no reason to allow an isolated practitioner to call himself a pain clinic. The diagnosis and management of patients with chronic pain has become so complex that multiple skills and knowledge are required. There are many possible combinations, but such a facility must have at least one physician who assumes responsibility for obtaining a complete history and performing a screening physical examination. Old records must also be reviewed. The specialty of the physician performing this review is not particularly relevant, but clearly someone with expertise in the type of disease process responsible for the patient's chronic pain should be either the referring physician or part of the pain treatment facility's assessment team. At least two other medical specialties as well as other types of health care providers should be represented to justify the term, multidisciplinary pain clinic. There is some question as to whether any pain management facilities which are not multidisciplinary should exist in a developed nation.

Other types of health care professionals are of great value in a pain treatment facility. These include psychologists, nurses, physical therapists, occupational therapists, social workers, vocational counselors and others. The variety and number will be determined by the types of patients seen and the number of visits per year to the facility. We should remember that the etiologies of chronic pain are not well understood; medical treatments have already failed many of these patients and effective evaluation and treatment may be administered by other health care professionals.

In summary, the developed nations should require that any facility calling itself a pain clinic or pain center offer a multidisciplinary array of diagnostic and treatment facilities. Single modality therapy programs should be identified by the modality they utilize; e.g., "Biofeedback Clinic" rather than the term "Pain Clinic." Neurosurgeons who perform pain-relieving procedures do not call themselves a "Pain Clinic," nor should any other solitary specialist. Health care facilities which specialize in one region of the body should be identified by that region in their title; e.g., "Headache Clinic," rather than "Pain Clinic." A Multi-disciplinary Pain Clinic or Center should provide comprehensive, integrated approaches to both assessment and treatment.

In developing nations, it may not be immediately possible to amass the professional and physical resources to establish a multidisciplinary pain clinic. A single health care provider may initiate a health care facility with the goals of adding other personnel as the institution evolves. This should be encouraged by IASP even though the health care facility at its inception may not meet the desired standards.

Pain Clinics and Pain Centers require not only physical resources but also specially trained health care providers. There is no specific training program in pain management at this time, so all health care providers have entered this area from existing specialties. Fellowships in pain management are beginning to develop, and those individuals who wish to specialize in pain management should be encouraged to obtain such a period of training. Others become reasonably skilled through their work with pain patients, but the field should move toward the establishment of specific training programs in pain management and the development of a method of evaluation and certification of individual health care providers by responsible leaders.

All pain clinics should work toward the use of a single method of coding diagnoses and treatments. Although the ICD-9 system is utilized in many countries, it is not particularly good for illnesses in which pain is the major complaint. The IASP Taxonomy system is a step in the right direction, but it will need further refinement before it becomes clinically acceptable. Nonetheless, excellence in pain management will require a standardized reporting system which can be used by all types of treatment facilities throughout the world.

Finally, excellence is dependent upon education of young health care providers who may wish to enter this field. Pain Centers need to establish educational programs on all levels to accomplish this goal. These programs should attempt to integrate with degree granting institutions in all the health sciences as well as post-graduate educational programs.

INDEX

205

Changing Your Address?

Make sure your subscription changes too! When you notify us of your new address, you can help make our job easier by including an exact copy of your Clinics label number with your old address (see illustration below.) This number identifies you to our computer system and will speed the processing of your address change. Please be sure this label number accompanies your old address and your corrected address—you can send an old Clinics label with your number on it or just copy it exactly and send it to the address listed below.

We appreciate your help in our attempt to give you continuous coverage. Thank you.

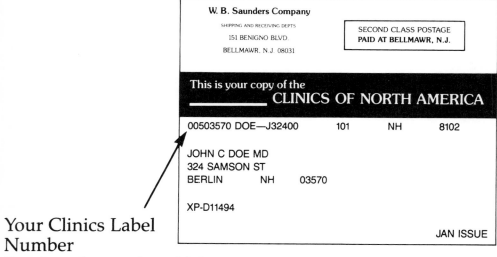

Your Clinics Label Number
Copy it exactly or send your label along with your address to:
W.B. Saunders Company, Customer Service
Orlando, FL 32887-4800
Call Toll Free 1-800-654-2452

Please allow four to six weeks for delivery of new subscriptions and for processing address changes.